Neurofibromatoses
in Clinical Practice

Rosalie E. Ferner · Susan M. Huson
D. Gareth R. Evans

Neurofibromatoses in Clinical Practice

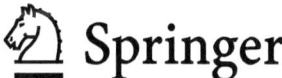 Springer

Authors

Rosalie E. Ferner, MD, FRCP
Consultant Neurologist
Department of Neurology
Guy's and St. Thomas' NHS
Foundation Trust London
and Department of Clinical
Neuroscience, Institute of
Psychiatry, King's College
London

Susan M. Huson, MD, FRCP
Consultant Clinical Geneticist
Manchester Academic Health
Science Centre
Saint Mary's Hospital
Manchester

D. Gareth R. Evans, MD, FRCP
Consultant Clinical Geneticist
Manchester Academic Health
Science Centre
Saint Mary's Hospital
Manchester

ISBN 978-0-85729-628-3   ISBN 978-0-85729-629-0 (eBook)
DOI 10.1007/978-0-85729-629-0
Springer London Dordrecht Heidelberg New York

British Library Cataloguing in Publication Data
A catalogue record for this book is available from the British Library

Library of Congress Control Number: 2011931682

Cover design: eStudioCalamar, Figueres/Berlin

Printed on acid-free paper

Springer is part of Springer Science+Business Media (www.springer.com)

Preface

Over the last 20 years there has been a rapid increase in our understanding of the disease mechanisms underlying neurofibromatosis 1 (NF1) and neurofibromatosis 2 (NF2), and related disorders. The neurofibromatoses are inherited diseases that involve the nervous system predominantly, but are distinct on both clinical and genetic grounds. Advances in molecular biology and mouse models have paved the way for clinical trials to combat benign and malignant tumors that characterize both diseases.

NF1 and NF2 are well documented in the medical literature, but partly due to the nomenclature, the distinction between the two conditions is blurred by clinicians. Furthermore the characterization of related and overlapping disorders has added to the complexity of diagnosis and management. The media has focused inexorably on people with NF1 who have extreme disfigurement, aiming to titillate rather than educate us, while NF2 is largely unknown outside of hospital practice.

In this book we aim to provide an accessible, up-to-date guide for nonspecialists on the diagnosis, management, and long-term care of people with NF1 and NF2. We emphasize the referral pathways to specialist centers for individuals with complex disease and highlight the available support networks. Above all we wish to show that coping with the neurofibromatoses relies on a partnership between patient and clinician, based on mutual trust and an ability to listen to the needs and choice of the individual.

Rosalie E. Ferner

Acknowledgments

We would like to thank all the people with Neurofibromatosis who have helped us with this book and contributed both pictures and personal reflections. We are very grateful to the National Commissioning Group for funding the specialist neurofibromatosis services. We would like to acknowledge our medical, nursing, and administrative colleagues and the members of the Neuro Foundation for their invaluable help and support in caring for individuals with neurofibromatosis 1 and 2.

Contents

Introduction

Rosalie E. Ferner

Definition of Neurofibromatosis 1 and Neurofibromatosis 2

Neurofibromatosis 1 (NF1) and neurofibromatosis 2 (NF2) are inherited neurocutaneous conditions that are clinically and genetically distinct and carry a high risk of tumor formation.[1] NF1 occurs in 1 in 2,500 births while NF2 is rare and has a birth incidence of 1 in 33,000.[2,3] NF1 and NF2 encode proteins that act as tumor suppressors by controlling cell growth and proliferation. The NF1 gene is on chromosome 17q11.2 and the protein product is neurofibromin; the gene for NF2 is on chromosome 22q 11.2 and encodes a protein known as merlin.[4-8] NF1 is characterized by café au lait patches, skin fold freckling, iris Lisch nodules, bony dysplasia, and benign peripheral nerve sheath tumors called neurofibromas.[9] The complications are variable, unpredictable, and widespread, ranging from learning difficulties, high blood pressure, and gastrointestinal symptoms to disfigurement and malignancy.[1]

Bilateral vestibular schwannomas are the hallmark lesion of NF2 and cause hearing and balance disturbances.[1,10] Schwannomas may develop on other cranial nerves, spinal nerve roots and peripheral nerves. Meningiomas, ependymomas and gliomas are associated with NF2.[1,10] Skin manifestations are less conspicuous than in NF1, but eye problems including juvenile cataracts are recognized.[1,10]

Recent Advances

Recent advances in molecular biology, mouse models of disease, and improvements in neuroimaging have permitted the distinction between NF1 and NF2 and the characterization of the many clinical manifestations.[1] They have resulted in the development of clinical trials that are underway to evaluate targeted therapy for disease complications. Conditions can be delineated that overlap with NF1 and NF2 but are distinct genetically and have different clinical outcomes. Legius syndrome is associated with mutations in the tumor suppressor gene *SPRED1* on chromosome 15, and is characterized by café au lait patches, freckling, and mild learning problems, without neurofibromas or Lisch nodules.[11] People with schwannomatosis have mutations in the *INI1/SMARCB1* tumor suppressor gene and develop multiple schwannomas in the absence of vestibular schwannomas or other NF2 tumors.[12,13]

Aims

Neurocutaneous diseases are complex to diagnose and treat and many patients require specialist multidisciplinary management and surveillance. However, due to multiple disease manifestations people with NF1 and NF2 present to different clinicians without specialist expertise in these diseases. Our aim is to provide a succinct accessible guide to the neurofibromatoses for the nonspecialist, including diagnosis, current management protocols, and indications for referral to specialist centers. The goal is optimum provision of care for neurocutaneous disease throughout the UK through partnership between local clinicians, specialist NF centers, and people with NF1 and NF2.

References

1. Ferner RE. Neurofibromatosis 1 and neurofibromatosis 2: a twenty first century perspective. *Lancet Neurol.* 2007;6:340-351.
2. Huson SM, Compston DAS, Clark P, et al. A genetic study of von Recklinghausen neurofibromatosis in south east Wales: prevalence, fitness, mutation rate and effect of parental transmission n severity. *J Med Genet.* 1989;26:704-711.
3. Evans DG, Howard E, Giblin C, et al. Birth incidence and prevalence of tumour prone syndromes: estimates from a UK genetic family register service. *Am J Med Genet.* 2010;15:327-332.
4. Viskochil D, Buchberg AN, Xu G, et al. Deletions and a translocation interrupt a cloned gene at the neurofibromatosis type 1 locus. *Cell.* 1990;62:1887-1892.
5. Wallace MR, Marchuk DA, Anderson LB, et al. Type 1 neurofibromatosis gene: identification of a larger transcript disrupted in three NG1 patients. *Science.* 1990;249:181-186.
6. Xu GF, O'Connell P, Viskochil D, et al. The neurofibromatosis type 1 gene encodes a protein related to GAP. *Cell.* 1990;62:599-608.
7. Rouleau GA, Merel P, Lutchman M, et al. Alteration in a new gene encoding a putative membrane-organizing protein causes neuro-fibromatosis type 2. *Nature.* 1993;363:515-521.
8. Troffater JA, MacCollin MM, Rutter JL, et al. A novel moesin-, ezrin-, radixin-like gene is a candidate for the neurofibromatosis 2 tumour suppressor. *Cell.* 1993;72:791-800.
9. National Institutes of Health Consensus Development Conference. Statement: neurofibromatosis. *Arch Neurol Chicago.* 1988;45:575-578.
10. Evans DGR, Huson S, Donnai D, et al. A clinical study of type 2 neurofibromatosis. *Q J Med.* 1992;84: 603-618.
11. Brems H, Chmara M, Sahbatou M, et al. Germline loss of function mutations in SPRED1 cause a neurofibromatosis 1 – like phenotype. *Nat Genet.* 2007;39:1120-1126.
12. MacCollin M, Chiocca EA, Evans DG, et al. Diagnostic criteria for Schwannomatosis. *Neurology.* 2005;64:1838-1845.
13. *INI1/SMARCB1* In familial Schwannomatosis. *Am J Med Genet.* 2007;80:805-810.

Chapter 1
Neurofibromatosis 1

Rosalie E. Ferner

- Neurofibromatosis 1(NF1) is a common autosomal dominant condition that primarily involves the skin and the nervous system.
- People with NF1 have an increased risk of developing benign and malignant tumors.

History of Current Terminology

Descriptions of people allegedly suffering from neurofibromatosis date back to the first century AD. One of the more convincing reports comes from Tilesius (1793) who depicted a short man with a curved spine and a large head.[1] An offensive smell was said to have emanated from multiple tumors on his body and Tilesius requested money from the public to assist him. The term "neurofibroma" was coined by Friedrich von Recklinghausen in 1882, when he described benign tumors forming on the peripheral nerve sheath and the disorder was named von Recklinghausen's disease in his honor.[2] International consensus groups started to meet in the late 1980s to collate information on clinical manifestations and pool genetic data. The current diagnostic criteria originate from the 1987 National Institutes of Health Consensus Development Conference who recommended that the disease be called neurofibromatosis 1 and proposed the diagnostic criteria for the condition (Table 1.1).[3]

R.E. Ferner et al., *Neurofibromatoses in Clinical Practice*,
DOI: 10.1007/978-0-85729-629-0_1,
© Springer-Verlag London Limited 2011

TABLE 1.1. Diagnostic criteria for NF.

The clinical diagnosis is made when at least two of the following are present[3]:

- A first degree relative with NF1
- Six or more café au lait patches >0.5 cm in children and >1.5 cm in adults
- Axillary or groin freckling
- Two or more neurofibromas of any type or one plexiform neurofibroma
- Two or more Lisch nodules (iris hamartomas)
- Optic pathway glioma
- Bony dysplasia of the sphenoid wing or
- Thinning of the long bone cortex with or without pseudarthrosis of the long bones[3]

Source: National Institutes of Health Consensus Development Conference Statement.[3] Copyright 1988 American Medical Association. All rights reserved

Epidemiology

NF1 has a birth frequency of 1 in 2,500–3,000 and a minimum prevalence of 1 in 4–5,000.[4] About half of people with NF1 have no family history of the disease and there are no asymptomatic carriers of NF1.[5]

Mosaic NF1

- Disease complications are uncommon in mosaic NF1
- The risk of passing on generalized NF1 to an offspring is low

This form of NF1 occurs in about 1 in 30,000 individuals and presents either as mild generalized disease that is clinically identical to NF1 or with segmental manifestations.[6] For instance, an individual might have café au lait patches, freckling, and neurofibromas localized to one body segment, but no other NF1 complications (Fig. 1.1).

Arrows show
neurofibromas

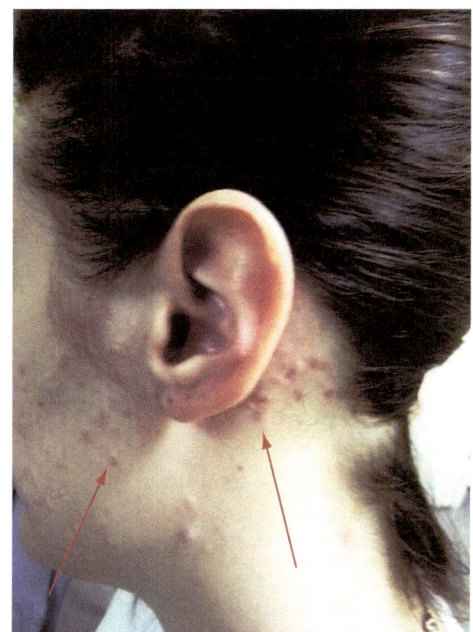

FIGURE 1.1. Segmental NF1. Cutaneous neurofibromas around the left side of the face and neck in individual with no other signs of NF1.

Genetics of NF1

In 1990 the *NF1* gene was identified on chromosome 17q11.2 and the protein product neurofibromin is found in high levels in the nervous system.[7-9] Neurofibromin decreases cell growth and proliferation by regulating the cellular proto-oncogene p21RAS and the serine threonine kinase MTOR (mammalian target of rapamycin).[8,10] People with NF1 are likely to develop benign and malignant tumors because neurofibromin loses its tumor suppressor function through gene mutation.

Genetics of Mosaic NF1

The *NF1* mutation arises in the egg or sperm *before* fertilization in classical generalized NF1 and *after* fertilization in mosaic

NF1.[6] The timing of the genetic change dictates how much of the body is involved in mosaic NF1. Mild generalized NF1 will develop from early mutations, whilst segmental disease results from mutations that occur later in formation of the embryo.[6]

Skin Manifestations of NF1

Skin problems are frequently the presenting manifestation of the disease and café au lait patches, freckling, and neurofibromas form part of the diagnostic criteria of NF1.[3]

Café au Lait Patches

Café au lait patches usually develop at birth or in early infancy and are observed in 99% of people with NF1 by age of 3 years (Fig. 1.2).[5,11] They have a smooth outline and may

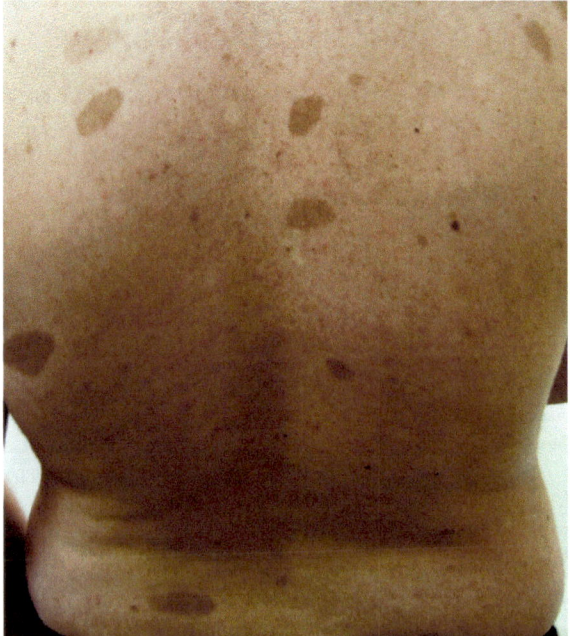

FIGURE 1.2. Multiple café au lait patches.

fade with age or be difficult to detect on pale skin or in patients with large numbers of neurofibromas. One or two café au lait patches are found in 10% of the general population and NF2 patients have café au lait patches in smaller numbers than in NF1.[5] It is important to remember that these skin manifestations are seen in overlapping conditions including Legius syndrome that has a milder course and does not have widespread complications (see Chap. 2).[12]

Freckling

Freckling is observed as hyperpigmented macules 1–3 mm in diameter in 85% of children after the age of 3 years.[5,11] It is found typically under the arms and in groins but is also found at the base of the neck, on the upper eyelids, over the trunk, and under the breasts (Fig. 1.3).[11]

Campbell de Morgan Spots

Campbell de Morgan spots are cherry red angiomas 1–3 mm in diameter and occur predominantly on the trunk and thighs (Fig. 1.4).[13] They are common in NF1 patients and develop at a younger age than in the general population.

Xanthogranulomas

Xanthogranulomas occur transiently in infancy as yellowish/orange nodules or papules and are noticeable as single or multiple lesions about 1 cm in diameter on the head, trunk, and limbs (Fig. 1.5).[14] A link between xanthogranulomas and the development of juvenile chronic myeloid leukemia has been suggested, but hematological screening is not warranted.[14]

Glomus Tumors

Glomus bodies control skin body temperature and individuals with glomus tumors present with pain around the nail bed

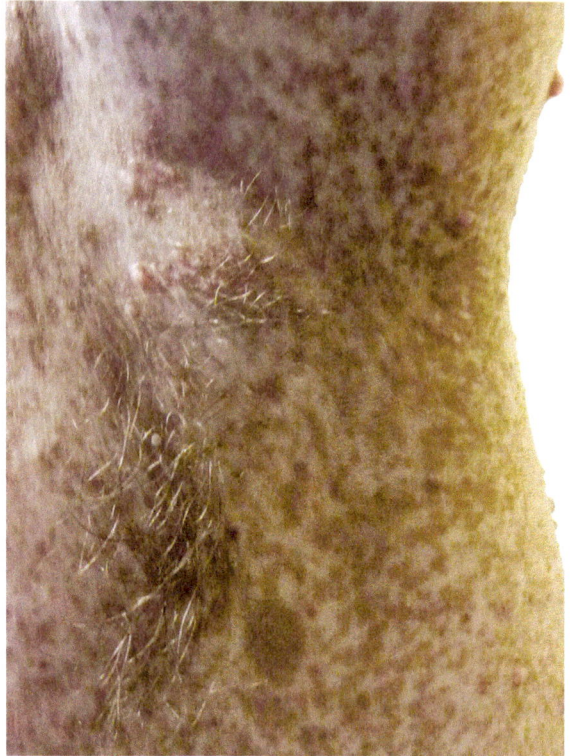

FIGURE 1.3. Axillary freckling.

of the fingers and toes.[15] The pain is precipitated by cold or by knocking the affected digit, and the pain is likened to being "hit by a hammer." Careful examination may reveal purplish discoloration around nail-bed that is exquisitely tender and the lesions may be multiple. MRI is helpful in locating the tumor and the pain is relieved by surgical removal of the glomus tumor.[15]

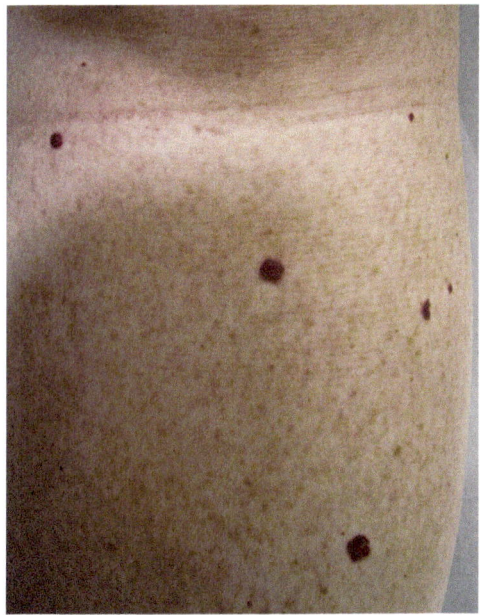

FIGURE 1.4. Campbell de Morgan spots (cutaneous angiomas) are associated with NF1.

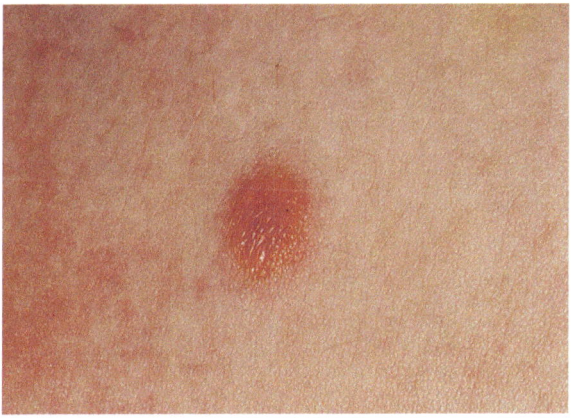

FIGURE 1.5. Xanthogranuloma in a young child with NF1 (Adapted from Ferner[5] with permission from Elsevier 2011).

Bone

- Pseudarthrosis of the long bone may present with spontaneous fracture and may be misinterpreted as non-accidental injury.
- Clinicians should be alert to this possibility, and examination of infant and parents is recommended to look for cutaneous signs of NF1.

Bone abnormalities are a source of major morbidity in NF1 and result from impaired maintenance of bone structure, bone overgrowth, and erosion by plexiform neurofibromas (Table 1.2).[16]

Pseudarthrosis of the Long Bones

Bowing of the long bone with thinning of the long bone cortex is evident in 2% of NF1 individuals in early infancy and principally affects the tibia, but involvement of the fibula, ulna, and radius is also reported (Fig. 1.6).[11,18] Fracture occurs spontaneously or after trivial injury and may be diagnosed wrongly as non-accidental injury. Prolonged delay in healing of the facture may result in formation of a false joint – a

TABLE 1.2. Types of bone problems and their frequency in NF1.

Bone manifestation[3,5,11,13,16,18-22]	Frequency (%)
Scoliosis	10
Scoliosis requiring surgery	5
Pseudarthrosis of the long bone	2
Scalloping of vertebral bodies	10
Sphenoid wing dysplasia	1
Non-ossifying fibromas	N/A
Short stature between 10th and 25th centile	30

FIGURE 1.6. Pseudarthrosis of the tibia in a young child with NF1 (Reproduced from Ferner[17] with permission from BMJ publishing group 2011).

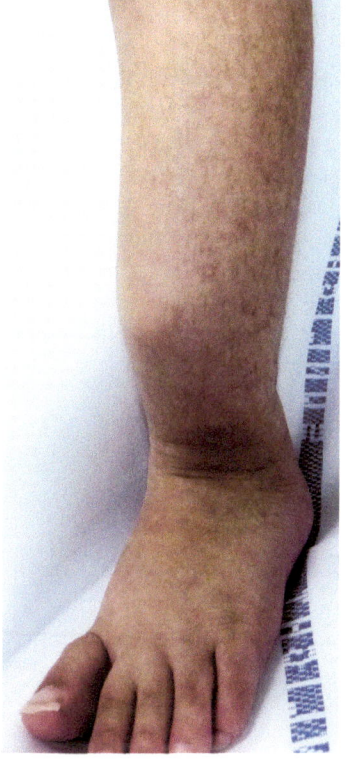

pseudarthrosis.[18] Clinical assessment and surgical treatment should be carried out by specialist orthopedics clinicians who have knowledge about the complexity of NF1 complications and the needs of the NF1 individual.

Short Stature

Short stature between the 10th and 25th centiles is present in a third of people with NF1 and involves the limbs and axial skeleton in proportion.[19] Rarely, NF1 children with tumors involving the hypothalamic pituitary axis present with small stature but routine neuroimaging is not required for all patients.

Reduced Bone Mineral Density

Reduction in bone mineral density has been described in about half of the individuals with NF1 but currently there are no data to confirm whether preventative treatment is warranted in every patient to reduce fracture.[20] Our practice is to assess clinical risk factors and to check 25 hydroxyvitamin D levels, parathyroid hormone levels, and bone chemistry in our patients, and to replace low levels of vitamin D. NF1 individuals with increased risk for osteoporosis should be referred to a metabolic bone unit for assessment of their treatment needs (see Table 1.3).[20]

TABLE 1.3. Risk factors for osteoporosis.

People with NF1 should be assessed for the risk factors for osteoporosis[19]:

- Female gender
- Family history of osteoporosis
- Late menarche
- Early menopause
- Injectable progesterone contraceptives
- Prolonged steroid treatment
- Anticonvulsant treatment
- Chronic disease – e.g. renal disease, liver disease, inflammatory bowel disease, celiac disease, hyperthyroidism, hyperparathyroidism, rheumatoid arthritis, anorexia nervosa
- Medical condition restricting mobility, e.g. multiple sclerosis
- Spinal instrumentation for scoliosis
- Low impact bone fracture
- Vertebral fracture
- Diet low in calcium
- History of smoking
- High alcohol consumption
- Low body mass index

Scoliosis

Scoliosis is diagnosed in about 10% of individuals with NF1 and presents as either the idiopathic or dystrophic form and most commonly affects the lower cervical and upper thoracic spine.[11,13,18] Dystrophic scoliosis does not usually develop before the age of 6 years and is uncommon after the first decade. A dystrophic curve typically involves 4–6 segments and causes distortion of the vertebral bodies and ribs. It may be caused by an underlying plexiform neurofibroma and occasionally is associated with respiratory compromise and rapid disease progression requiring surgical intervention with spinal fusion.[18] Yearly assessment of the spine should be undertaken until adulthood and children who develop scoliosis should be referred to a specialist spinal unit for monitoring.[13]

Non-ossifying Neurofibromas

These benign lesions of the tubular long bones should be distinguished from malignant tumors. They are usually asymptomatic but patients may complain of pain and infrequently they are associated with pathological fracture.[21]

Vertebral Scalloping

Vertebral scalloping is an exaggerated concavity of dorsal aspect of the vertebra, and posterior vertebral scalloping is a common radiological finding in NF1. It may be associated with scoliosis or with and a plexiform neurofibroma.[22]

Neurological Complications of NF1

Neurological complications are an important source of morbidity and mortality in NF1 and the commonest manifestation is mild cognitive impairment. Neurofibromas are the hallmark lesion of NF1 and cause neurological deficit by pressure on peripheral nerves, spinal nerve roots, and the spinal cord. Neurological sequelae may result from tumors and malformations, cerebrovascular disease, epilepsy, and as a secondary consequence of bony deformities of the skull and spine (Table 1.4).[5]

TABLE 1.4. Manifestations of NF1 in the peripheral and central nervous system.[5]

Peripheral nerve

- Neurofibromas – subcutaneous, plexiform[a]
- Malignant peripheral nerve sheath tumors
- Neurofibromatous neuropathy

Spinal canal

- Neurofibromas – spinal nerve root[a]
- Spinal tumor – glioma
- Secondary consequence of scoliosis

Brain

- Cognitive impairment[a]
- Epilepsy
- Cerebrovascular disease
- Multiple sclerosis

Brain and optic pathway tumors

- Glioma
- Optic pathway glioma[a]
- T2 hyperintensities on MRI[a]

Malformations/consequence of skull deformity

- Chiari 1 malformation
- Aqueduct stenosis
- Sphenoid wing dysplasia
- Macrocephaly[a]

[a]Denotes common neurological features

Neurofibromas

Classification of Neurofibromas

The Schwann cell is the predominant cell in a neurofibroma, but this benign peripheral nerve sheath tumor also contains fibroblasts, perineurial cells, and axons in an extracellular

TABLE 1.5. Neurofibromas and their potential to cause cosmetic problems, neurological deficit, and malignant change[5].

Neurofibroma type	Cosmetic problems	Neurology deficit	Malignant change
Cutaneous	++	0	0
Subcutaneous	±	+	+
Plexiform	++	++	++
Spinal nerve root	0	++	++

++ = very frequent, + = frequent, ± = occasional, 0 = never

matrix.[23] There are different forms of neurofibroma, and it is imperative to recognize the neurofibroma types that are likely to cause significant cosmetic problems, neurological deficit, or undergo malignant change (Table 1.5).[5]

Cutaneous Neurofibromas

Cutaneous neurofibromas develop in 99% of NF1 patients, usually in the late teens and early twenties, but occasionally in childhood (Fig. 1.7).[11,13] They increase in size and number during pregnancy but hormonal contraceptives do not appear to influence growth and are not contraindicated.[5,24] Neurofibromas are soft lesions, sometimes have a purplish tinge, and are the source of significant psychological problems because of their appearance. Stinging and itching are common symptoms; the latter does not respond to antihistamines, but emollients and avoidance of very warm environments may be helpful. Local excision is the treatment of choice, but patients should be informed that there is a risk of a thickened scar and plastic surgeons should remove lesions on the face or neck to get the best possible cosmetic result. Laser is useful for some small neurofibromas, but is not suitable for removal of very large numbers of tumors.[13]

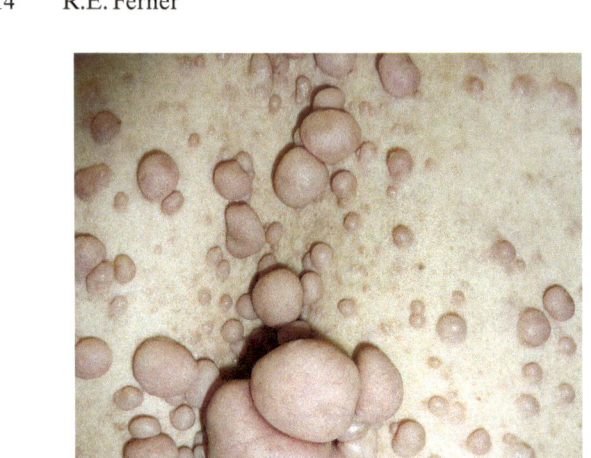

FIGURE 1.7. Multiple cutaneous neurofibromas on the back.

Subcutaneous Neurofibromas and Differential Diagnosis

- It is important to distinguish subcutaneous neurofibromas from other subcutaneous tumors that have different clinical outcomes and management requirements.
- Clinical examination and imaging may not be sufficient and histology is frequently required to confirm the diagnosis.

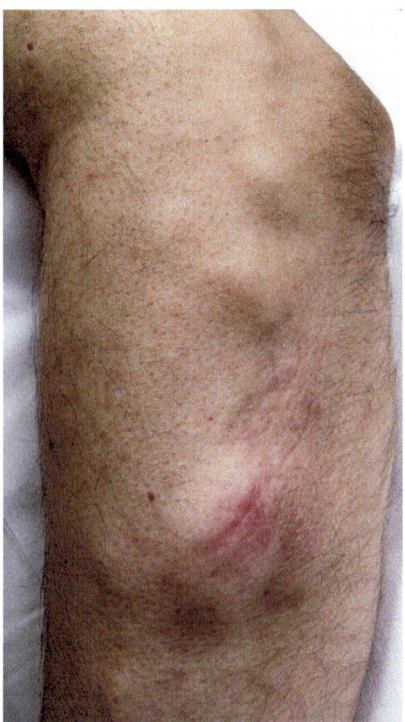

FIGURE 1.8. Subcutaneous neurofibromas on upper limb (Reproduced from Ferner[17] with permission from BMJ publishing group 2011).

Subcutaneous neurofibromas are firm lesions that form under the skin and frequently give rise to pain, tingling, numbness, and weakness (Fig. 1.8).[5,11] It is essential to distinguish subcutaneous neurofibromas from schwannomas as the latter have a different clinical course from neurofibromas. Schwannomas are peripheral nerve sheath tumors composed solely of Schwann cells, and unlike subcutaneous neurofibromas only very rarely undergo malignant change.[5] They may occur as single sporadic tumors but are cardinal features of NF2 and Schwannomatosis.[25,26] Excision or biopsy and histology is the only way to be certain of the diagnosis as neurofibromas are often similar to schwannomas clinically and on magnetic resonance imaging (MRI). Individuals who present with subcutaneous lumps on the trunk, distal arms, and proximal thighs in the absence of neurological deficit or other NF1 manifestations are likely to have multiple lipomas. Some patients with Legius syndrome have been reported to have lipomas.[12] Ultrasound may be helpful in distinguishing lipomas from nerve sheath tumors but excision and histology may be advisable in some cases (see Chaps. 2 and 3).[5,11] People who develop subcutaneous breast lumps should be referred to a breast unit as breast carcinoma cannot be distinguished reliably from a neurofibroma. It is important to note that there is an 8% cumulative risk of developing breast cancer before the age of 50 years in women with NF1, compared with 2% in the general population.[27] The symptoms from glomus tumors may be attributed erroneously to pain from a subcutaneous neurofibroma and clinicians should be alert to this possibility when symptoms arise in the fingers or toes.[15]

Spinal Neurofibromas

Neurofibromas may form at all levels on the spinal nerve roots and in many people are asymptomatic. However, some neurofibromas cause pressure on the spinal nerve root or spinal cord and may present with pain, sensory symptoms, bladder or bowel disturbance, sexual dysfunction, or motor deficit, which occasionally requires surgical intervention (Figs. 1.9 and 1.10). The degree of cord compression on neuroimaging does not always accord with the neurological deficit and the need for surgical intervention should be determined by clinicians who are conversant with cord compression in neurofibromatosis 1.[5,28]

Plexiform Neurofibromas

Benign plexiform neurofibromas may cause pain, neurological deficit, respiratory impairment, sphincter disturbance hemorrhage, infection, and disfigurement.

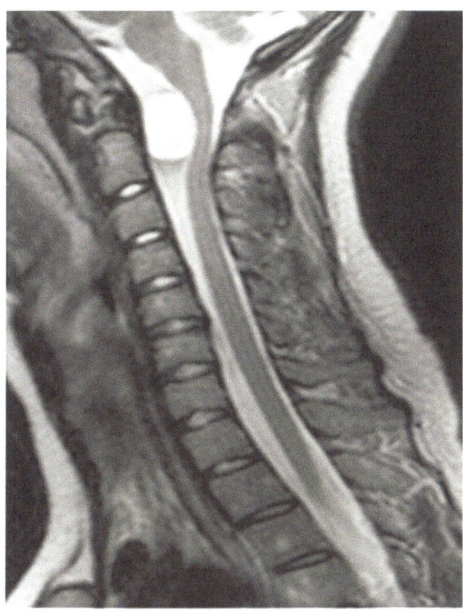

FIGURE 1.9. Cord compression in NF1 patient present with progressive limb weakness. Neurofibromas cause marked cord compression and narrowing particularly at C1–2 and C4, C5–6.

Plexiform neurofibromas form either as nodular lesions that are confined to the nerve or develop as diffuse tumors that grow along the length of the nerve and involve multiple nerve branches (Fig. 1.11).[5,11,13] Impingement on surrounding soft tissue and underlying bone hypertrophy are associated with extensive tumors (Fig. 1.12). Superficial neurofibromas may be accompanied by skin thickening, hair growth, and hyper-pigmentation (Fig. 1.13).[5,11,13]

Plexiform neurofibromas are thought to be congenital in origin and are detected clinically in a third of NF1 individuals.[11] Newer imaging techniques with whole body MRI reveal internal neurofibromas in over half of people with NF1,[29] but some deep-seated tumors can remain quiescent

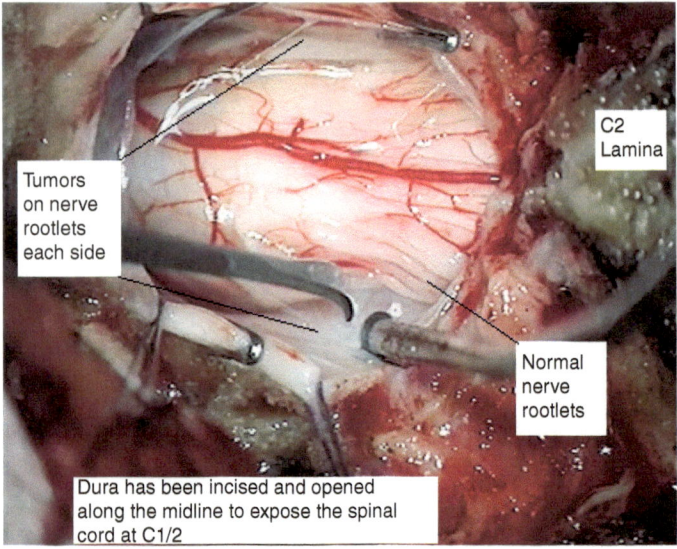

FIGURE 1.10. Neurofibromas causing cord compression at C1–2 (slide from Mr. Walsh consultant neurosurgeon King's College Hospital, London).

for long periods of time (Fig. 1.14). However, benign plexiform neurofibromas are a source of major morbidity due to their unsightly appearance and potential to cause neurological symptoms and deficit, bowel and bladder disturbance, obstructive sleep apnea, restrictive lung disease, life-threatening hemorrhage, and delayed wound healing.[5,11,13]

Surgery should be undertaken only in specialist units that are conversant with the possible complications of neurofibroma surgery. Novel therapies that aim to reduce neurofibroma growth and restore the tumor suppressor function are still at the clinical trial stage. Pain arising from neurofibromas usually responds to a combination of amitryptyline and gabapentin or pregabalin.

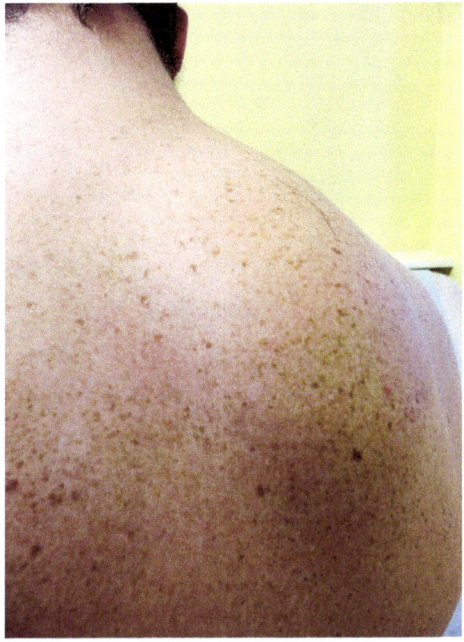

FIGURE 1.11. Nodular plexiform neurofibroma on the back of a NF1 individual.

Malignant Peripheral Nerve Sheath Tumor

- Urgent referral to a specialist unit is advocated if a diagnosis of malignant peripheral nerve sheath tumor is suspected. Symptoms that indicate potential malignant change in a neurofibroma include one or more of the following:
- Persistent or nocturnal pain
- Hard texture
- Rapid growth
- New or unexplained neurological deficit

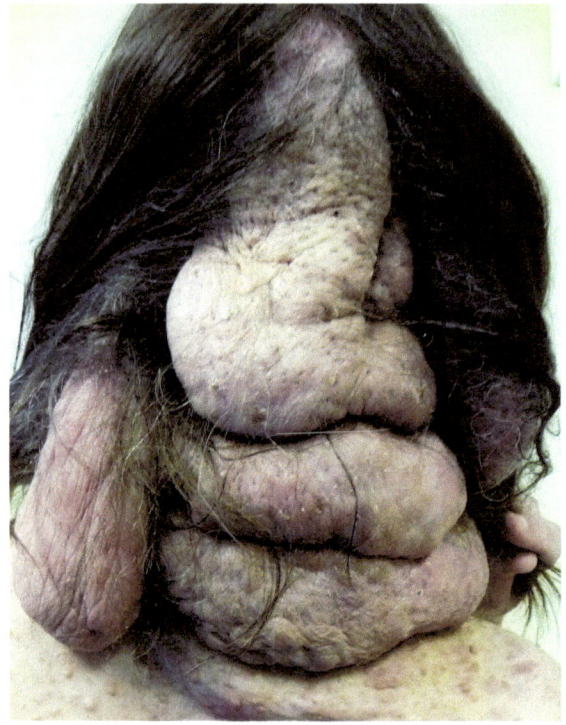

FIGURE 1.12. Very extensive plexiform neurofibroma involving the posterior neck and scalp. Surgery produced marked cosmetic improvement.

People with NF1 have about a 10% life-time risk of developing malignant peripheral nerve sheath tumor (MPNST)[30]; the tumors usually occur in the second or third decades although they also develop less frequently in young children and in the elderly.[31] High-grade MPNSTs metastasize widely and have a poor prognosis, but low-grade tumors that are diagnosed early and treated appropriately are compatible with long-term survival (Fig. 1.15). The tumor usually arises in a benign plexiform neurofibroma but occasionally may develop without a known preexisting neurofibroma.[31]

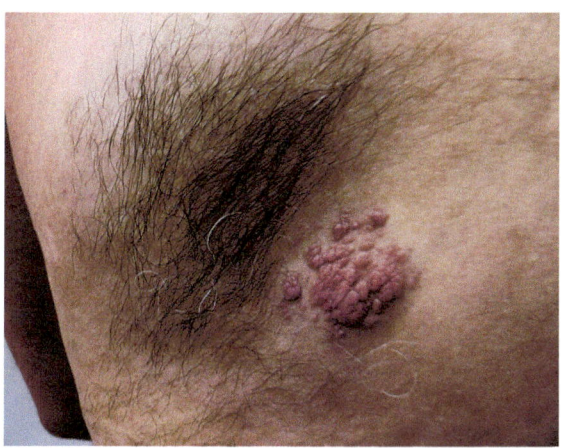

FIGURE 1.13. Superficial plexiform neurofibroma with skin thickening and hair growth.

Diagnosis of MPNST

MPNST is difficult to diagnose as the occurrence of a lump is not unusual in individuals who have multiple neurofibromas on and under the skin.[31] The symptoms of a benign neurofibroma overlap with MPNST or are misinterpreted as rheumatological or orthopedic problems. Clinicians should have a low threshold for investigating NF1 patients who present with symptoms arising in the cervical nerve roots or that are suggestive of sciatica.

MRI shows the site and extent of the tumor but does not reliably diagnose malignancy. [18][F] 2-fluoro-2-deoxy-D-glucose positron emission tomography–computerized tomography with delayed imaging and targeted biopsy is the most sensitive and specific method of diagnosing MPNST within the context of NF1.[32] Patients with suspected malignancy should be referred urgently to one of the nationally commissioned neurofibromatosis units for assessment and management.

Treatment of MPNST

The aim of treatment is complete removal of the tumor with tumor-free margins. Radiotherapy is given for incompletely

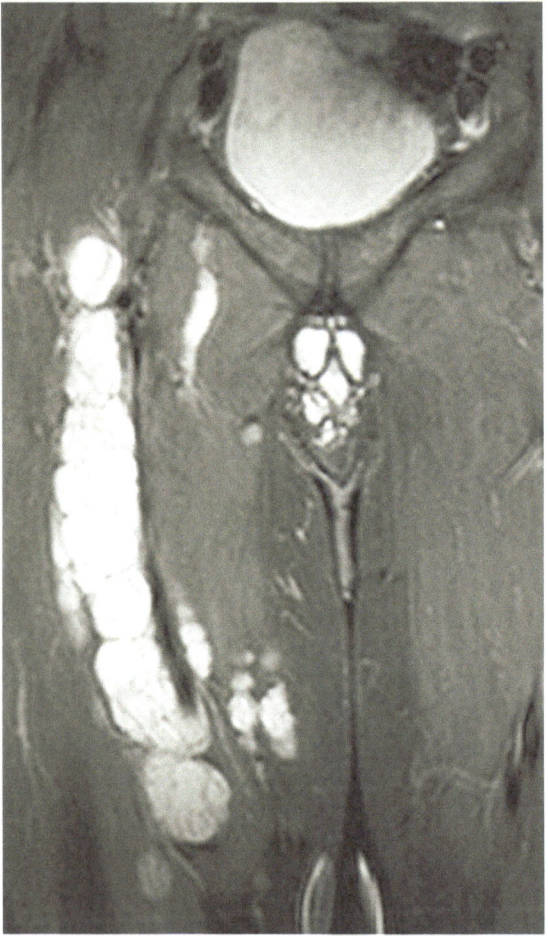

FIGURE 1.14. Deep-seated plexiform neurofibroma involving pelvis and thigh as manifestation of mosaic NF1.

excised lesions and for high-grade tumors and chemotherapy with doxorubicin and ifosfamide is administered for wide-spread disease as palliation.[31]

Increased surveillance is recommended for NF1 individuals with increased risk for developing MPNST. These include people with a microdeletion of the *NF1* gene; patients who have had prior radiotherapy or malignancy or a family

Arrows show malignant
peripheral nerve sheath
tumor in the neck in
parapharyngeal region

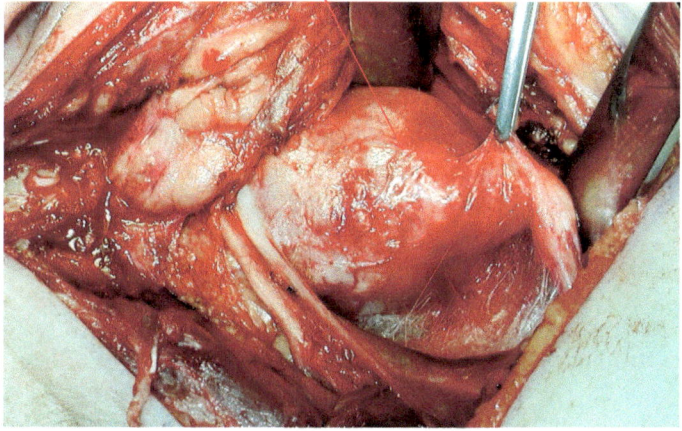

FIGURE 1.15. Parapharyngeal malignant peripheral nerve sheath tumor in patient presenting with painful, enlarging, neck lump. (Slide courtesy of Michael Gleeson, Guy's and St. Thomas' NHS Foundation Trust).

history of cancer; a diagnosis of neurofibromatous neuropathy; deep-seated neurofibromas; and neurofibromas involving the brachial and lumbosacral plexus.[31]

Neurofibromatous Neuropathy

About 1% of NF1 adults develop a symmetrical axonal neuropathy that is associated with thickened peripheral nerves due to infiltration by neurofibromatous tissue.[33] The neuropathy is not progressive and patients may be asymptomatic or report mild sensory or motor symptoms. Examination may reveal distal weakness, retained or reduced reflexes, and sensory findings include impairment of light touch, pain sensation, or loss of vibration sense. The diagnosis is confirmed on neurophysiology and common causes of axonal neuropathy such as diabetes mellitus should be excluded. People with neurofibromatous neuropathy require careful monitoring because of the increased risk of developing MPNST.[33]

Cognitive Impairment

Cognitive impairment in NF1 is characterized by a lowering of IQ, specific learning problems, and behavioral difficulties.[34] People with NF1 may display superior academic ability, 4–6% have significant intellectual handicap (IQ < 70), and the majority have an IQ in the low average range.[34]

Specific Learning Problems

At least 60% of NF1 children are diagnosed with specific learning problems and males and females are affected equally. They experience difficulty with visual spatial tasks, memory and language skills, which may lead to underachievement in reading, writing, and mathematics.[34] Children may exhibit poor planning, time management, and organizational ability, and failure to absorb and integrate new information leads to unstructured and untidy classwork.[34] Incoordination and joint laxity may prevent NF1 individuals from riding a bike, tying shoelaces, or holding a pen correctly.

Behavioral Problems

Behavioral problems manifest as attention deficit hyperactivity disorder, sleep disturbance, impulsive temperament, inability to understand nonverbal cues, social immaturity, and isolation. Autistic spectrum disorder has been reported in NF1 patients.[5,34]

Management of Learning Problems in NF1

Early recognition of cognitive impairment is essential, so that the child may receive appropriate assessment and support at school. Close liaison between the parent, school, and community pediatrician is of paramount importance. Children with attention problems respond to judicious treatment with methylphenidate and occupational therapy is helpful for coordination difficulties.[13,34]

Novel Therapy for Cognitive Problems in NF1

An *Nf1* mouse model has demonstrated that learning problems in mice respond to a reduction in p21ras activity.[35] Lovostatin reverses p21ras activity and initial clinical trials of statins in children with NF1 have shown a good safety profile.[36] Longer therapeutic trials are being undertaken to determine the efficacy of the drugs in NF1 children with cognitive problems.

Brain Tumors

The following may indicate signs of raised intracranial pressure and require prompt assessment if the symptoms are unexplained:

- Early morning headache and vomiting
- Visual disturbance
- Alteration in consciousness

Gliomas

The main tumor type in NF1 is the glioma and it is located predominantly in the optic pathway and brainstem.[5,13] Most tumors are low-grade pilocytic astrocytomas and frequently are asymptomatic, but some lesions have an aggressive course (Fig. 1.16).[5] Patients who present with symptomatic gliomas in adulthood or with tumors that are outside the optic pathway have a less favorable outcome.[37] Many gliomas do not require treatment but progressive symptoms and deficit require neurosurgical assessment and treatment options include surgery, radiotherapy, and chemotherapy.[5] Meningiomas are characteristic of NF2 and any occurrence in NF1 patients is coincidental.

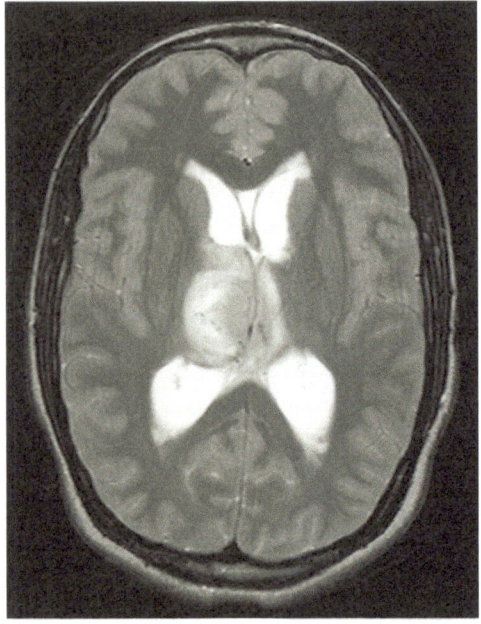

FIGURE 1.16. Young patient with NF1 who presented with early morning headache due to raised intracranial pressure from a high-grade thalamic glioma.

T2 Hyperintensities on Brain MRI

T2 hyperintensities (formally termed UBOs or unidentified bright objects) are visible on brain MRI in the majority of children with NF1 particularly in the basal ganglia, brainstem, and cerebellum (Fig. 1.17).[34,38] They are distinguished readily from brain tumors as they do not cause symptoms or neurological deficit and do not produce mass effect and distortion of brain tissue. Serial neuroimaging demonstrates that most lesions disappear in early adulthood and probably they represent delayed myelination or gliosis. Initially, they were thought to be related to the presence of cognitive impairment, but there has been no consistent conclusion among researchers.[34] However, lesions in thalamus appear to be associated with severe generalized cognitive difficulties.[39]

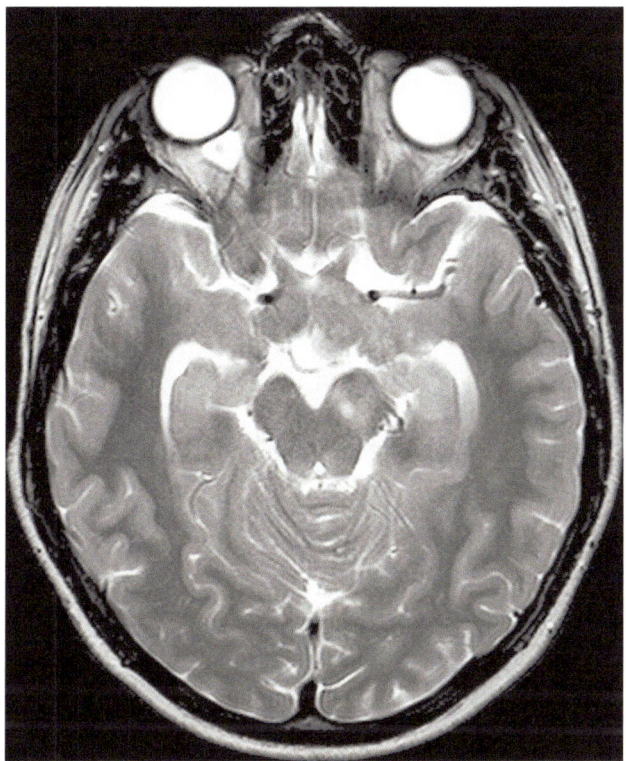

FIGURE 1.17. T2 hyperintensity (formerly known as unidentified bright object) on brain MRI in young child which did not cause symptoms or neurological deficit.

Optic Pathway Gliomas (OPG)

- Young children do not complain of visual loss.
- Children with NF1 require yearly visual screening for OPG until at least age 7 years.
- Screening for OPG with brain MRI is not warranted in asymptomatic children.
- CT brain scans should not be performed in young children with NF1 to avoid unnecessary radiation.

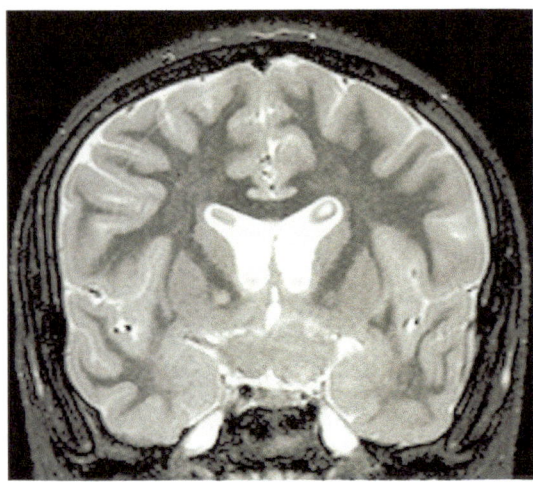

FIGURE 1.18. Optic pathway glioma involving optic chiasm in child who presented with progressive decline in visual acuity.

Presentation of NF1-OPG and Difference from Sporadic OPG

OPG are found in 15% of NF1 children but only about 5–7% ever cause symptoms (Fig. 1.18).[40] Sporadic OPG are biologically different from NF1-associated tumors, they are more likely to present with raised intracranial pressure and hydrocephalus and have a worse visual outcome with higher morbidity and mortality.[40] The greatest risk for developing NF1-OPG is under the age of 7 years and the mean age at diagnosis is about 4 years.[40] Rarely, new OPG can develop or progress in older children or adults, but only eight such patients were detected in three large NF1 centers.[41]

Signs and Symptoms of NF1-OPG

A thorny problem in detecting NF1-OPG is that young children do not complain of visual loss and may have significant visual problems before the diagnosis is made. Visual signs are present in about 60% of NF1 children with OPG and include reduced visual acuity, propotosis, squint, abnormal pupil responses, impaired visual fields and color vision, pale or swollen optic disc, and precocious puberty.[40] The latter usually occurs in children over 6 years and the initial sign of accelerated linear growth may indicate that the OPG is involving the pituitary or hypothalamus.

Screening for OPG

There is no indication for screening all NF1 children with brain MRI as the majority of the tumors detected will not require treatment and radiological progression does not always go hand in hand with visual deterioration.[40] There may be a role for neuroimaging when no useful visual assessment can be obtained from a child but this should be performed only in specialist centers. Changes on serial visual evoked potentials are difficult to interpret clinically and may not correlate with visual impairment.[40] OPG is the commonest non-refractive cause of visual impairment in NF1 and the aim of age-appropriate visual acuity assessment is to detect abnormalities in visual function that are caused by OPG. The current recommendation is to perform visual screening in children with NF1 at least annually until the age of 7 years and every 2 years thereafter until 18 years.[13,40] There are no specific recommendations for adults but they are encouraged to have a visual assessment every 2 years.

Visual acuity assessment is the most useful detection method for OPG and color vision impairment, nystagmus and squint are usually associated with visual acuity loss when due to NF1 OPG.[40] Visual field abnormalities are almost always accompanied by reduction in visual acuity and assessment of visual fields is frequently unreliable in young children and particularly in patients with learning problems.

Surveillance of a Child with Known NF1-OPG

There is debate about the optimum surveillance of a child with OPG but the frequency of visual assessments and MRI will depend on the site of the tumor, the degree of visual impairment and other symptoms, as well as evidence of progressive disease. Initially, assessments may be undertaken every 3 months and decrease to yearly if there is stable disease.[40]

Indications for Treatment of NF1-OPG

Opinions have varied in different units on the indications for starting treatment in children with NF1-OPG. However, there is agreement that children should be referred for treatment if there is progressive decline in visual acuity of two lines or more (on an age appropriate visual test) in combination with tumor progression on MRI.[40] Reduced vision in one eye and risk to vision in the other eye, severe visual impairment at diagnosis, progressive proptosis, and precocious puberty may also prompt initiation of treatment.[40]

Treatment for NF1-OPG

Radiotherapy is contraindicated for OPG in NF1 children because of the high risk of second malignancies, either glioma or MPNST.[42] Moreover, endocrine problems, cerebrovascular disease, and neuropsychological difficulties may occur in children who have been treated with radiotherapy. Surgery may be undertaken for large orbital tumors with no useful vision, for cosmetic reasons, or to treat corneal exposure.[40] Tumors with an unusual presentation or location may require biopsy and surgery is carried out to reduce tumor bulk of some hypothalamic or chiasm OPGs. The mainstay of treatment for NF1-OPG is chemotherapy with carboplatin and vincristine, which have been shown to improve vision and to result in reduction of tumor size.[43] There is no consistent second-line therapy, but the mTOR inhibitor (see section on NF1 Genetics) rapamycin has been advocated as a novel therapy because it reduces astrocyte growth and might have a role in controlling OPG tumor growth.[44]

Nervous System Malformations

Macrocephaly with a head circumference above the 98th centile is present in about 45% of NF1 patients but is not related to cognitive impairment.[11,13] Aqueduct stenosis causing hydrocephalus and symptoms of raised intracranial pressure is present in about 1.5% of patients and some require surgical correction.[5,11] Chiari 1 malformation has been reported in NF1 and occurs when the cerebellar tonsils herniate downward, occasionally causing occipital headache worse on exertion or cerebellar symptoms.[5,11] An absent sphenoid wing is diagnostic of NF1 and affects 1% of people with NF1.[3,5,11] The contents of the temporal lobe are pushed through to the orbit resulting in pulsating exophthalmus but vision is not compromised and surgical correction is rarely warranted (Fig. 1.19).

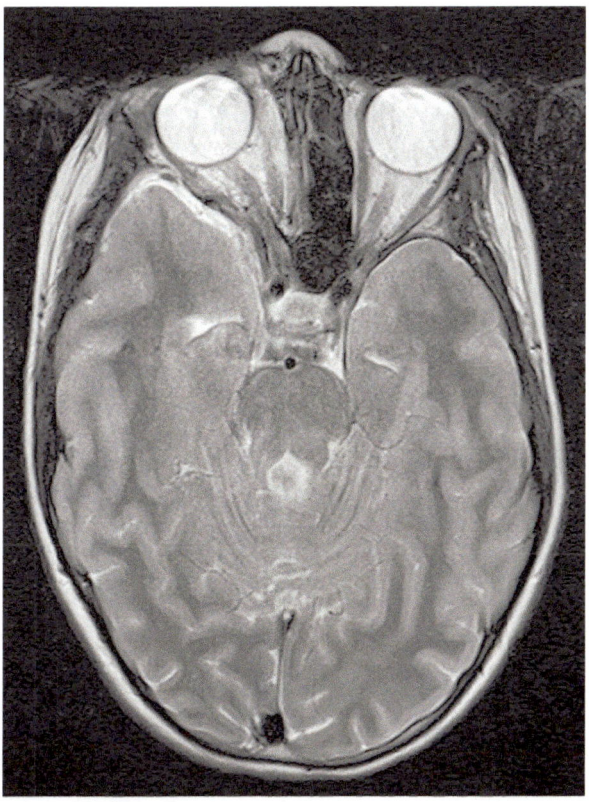

FIGURE 1.19. An absent sphenoid wing causes herniation of the temporal lobe into the orbit and proptosis of the right eye.

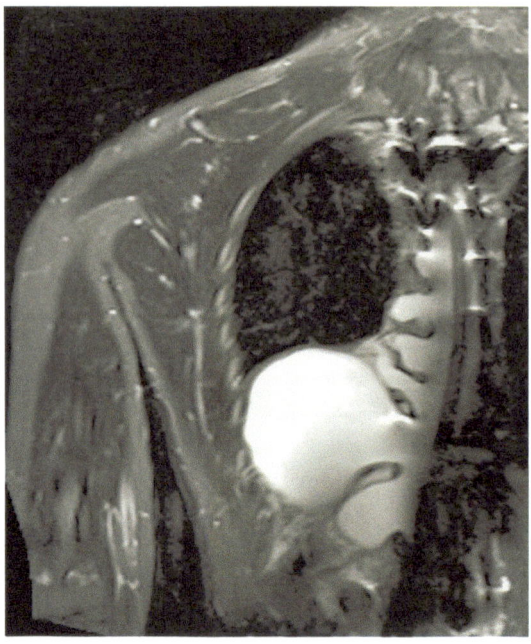

FIGURE 1.20. Dural ectasia (expansion) in thoracic spine in NF1 patient with back pain.

Dural ectasia is an outpouching of the dural sac and is recognized in association with NF1 (Fig. 1.20).[45] It may be an asymptomatic neuroradiological finding but sometimes causes pain or neurological deficit.

Epilepsy

Epilepsy is reported in about 6–7% of NF1 individuals and may be associated with an underlying cortical dysplasia.[46] The onset of seizures is observed from early infancy to late middle age and all seizure types have been reported with a preponderance of focal epilepsy.[5,11,46] Most patients achieve good seizure control, but clinicians should be aware of the increased risk of osteoporosis in NF1 when prescribing anti-convulsants (see section on osteoporosis), and levetiracetam should be used cautiously in people with learning difficulties because of the risk of deteriorating behavior.

Multiple Sclerosis

Relapsing remitting and primary progressive multiple sclero-sis may be observed with increased frequency in people with NF1 and immunosuppressant therapy for multiple sclerosis should be instituted with care, because NF1 is a tumor sup-pressor condition.[47] However, there have been no reported cases of malignancy in NF1 patients who have received immunosuppression for multiple sclerosis. Individuals with NF1 and multiple sclerosis may present a diagnostic dilemma if they present with upper motor neurone signs in the limbs, but MRI will differentiate demyelination from deficit caused by spinal neurofibromas.

Cerebrovascular Disease

Neurovascular disturbances occur in 6% of NF1 children on neuroimaging and are associated with intrinsic abnormalities of intracranial blood vessels.[48] Stenosis and/or occlusion of the internal carotid and cerebral arteries has been docu-mented and cerebral aneurysm and moyamoya disease are associated with NF1.[49] Patients have an increased risk of hypertension, which is in turn a risk factor for both cerebral hemorrhage and infarction. It has been suggested that cere-brovascular disease is an important cause of early death in NF1 individuals but this has not been corroborated in our experience in three large NF centers over a 20 year period.[50] Nonetheless, clinicians should have a low threshold for investigating patients who present with symptoms or signs suggestive of cerebrovascular disease and assiduous management of risk factors is essential including hypertension, heart disease, diabetes mellitus, high cholesterol, polycythemia, thromboembolic disease, and smoking.

The Eye (See Section on Neurological Complications for Optic Pathway Glioma)

In 1937, the Austrian ophthalmologist Karl Lisch visualized dome-shaped pigmented hamartomas of the iris in three patients.[51] Lisch nodules do not cause symptoms, but are pathognomic of NF1 and slit-lamp examination confirms their presence in virtually all adults with the disease (Fig. 1.21). Choroidal abnormalities, congenital and acquired glaucoma have been reported in association with NF1.[5] Neurofibromas on the eyelid may obstruct vision and occasionally require intervention from an oculoplastic surgeon. Idiopathic unilateral or bilateral ptosis has been observed in NF1, but other causes should be excluded including thyroid disease and neuromuscular problems.

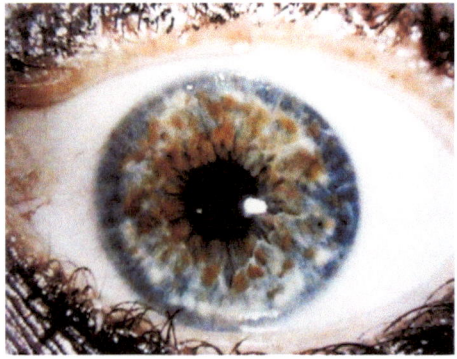

FIGURE 1.21. Lisch nodules (dome-shaped hamartomas) on the iris of NF1 patient.

Cardiovascular Disease

Hypertension

- Blood pressure requires lifelong monitoring in NF1
- Hypertension develops with increased frequency and may be idiopathic or be associated with renal artery stenosis or pheochromocytoma.
- Idiopathic hypertension is managed in the same way as in the general population

Renal Artery Stenosis

Renal artery stenosis is diagnosed in about 2% of NF1 individuals and is most commonly related to a fibromuscular dysplasia of the major or small renal vessels.[11,13,52] Aneurysm formation is detected in about 30% of cases and rarely renal artery stenosis may be the result of compression from an adjacent tumor.[13,52] The complication should be considered in a hypertensive child, pregnant women who present with high blood pressure, and in older individuals with poorly controlled hypertension. Investigation is undertaken by specialist renal units and treatment includes antihypertensive medication, transluminal angioplasty, and surgery.[13]

Pheochromocytoma

NF1-related pheochromocytoma is diagnosed in 2% of patients; the adrenal medulla is the commonest site and duodenal carcinoid has been reported as a concomitant finding.[5,13,53] Pheochromocytoma may be bilateral and 12% of tumors are malignant. Palpitations, headache, sweating or dizziness, and sustained or intermittent hypertension are characteristic features. However, the symptoms may be confused with anxiety, and the NF1 patient group is difficult to assess in this regard because the burden of disease causes psychological problems. Clinicians should be alert to the possibility that pheochromocytomas may cause severe hypertension leading to life-threatening cardiovascular compromise, particularly during surgery or pregnancy. Measurement of 24-h urinary catecholamines should be undertaken in individuals with unexplained hypertension or associated clinical manifestations. It is important to ask patients to start the collection during the symptomatic period if the symptoms are intermittent. Alternative diagnostic techniques should be undertaken by specialist centers if there is clinical suspicion of a pheochromocytoma and the 24-h urinary catecholamines are normal. The aim is surgical excision of the tumor with prior alpha and beta blockade to prevent fluctuations in blood pressure and cardiac arrhythmias.[13,53]

Heart Disease

Pulmonary stenosis is the commonest manifestation of congenital heart disease that is documented in 2% of NF1 individuals.[5,13,50] Children with unexplained cardiac murmurs require cardiological assessment and echocardiography. Cardiovascular symptoms may arise from coarctation and aneurysm of the aorta or from compression from mediastinal neurofibromas.[50] Coarctation of the aorta can be detected by measuring the blood pressure in the arms and legs. Although cardiovascular disease is purported to be a major cause of death in young people in NF1, this has not been substantiated in the large NF1 patient centers in England.[50]

Respiratory Problems

People with severe scoliosis and with high cord compression due to plexiform neurofibromas need formal respiratory evaluation to exclude restrictive lung disease. High-grade malignant peripheral nerve sheath tumors spread to the lung causing shortness of breath or nonproductive cough. We have also encountered NF1 patients with primary lung cancer and with lung metastases from breast cancer.

Gastrointestinal Disease

Gastrointestinal Stromal Tumor GIST

The link between mesenchymal gastrointestinal stromal tumors (GIST) and NF1 is well established and these tumors have been reported in 7% of NF1[54] individuals. They are located mostly in the small bowel and may be multiple. Symptoms include abdominal pain, anemia, and upper or lower gastrointestinal bleeding. The tumors need to be distinguished from malignant peripheral nerve sheath tumors as the clinical manifestations are similar and both are positive on 18FDG PET CT. GIST usually require surgical excision and clinical monitoring, treatment with imatinib is being evaluated and the outcome in NF1-associated GIST is usually good.

Carcinoid Tumors

Carcinoid tumors are found preferentially in the duodenum in NF1 patients and may be associated with a pheochromocytoma.[11,55] The clinical manifestations include facial flushing and telangiectasia, diarrhea, and wheezing. The diagnosis is made by increased levels of the serotonin metabolite, urinary 5-hydroxy-indoleacetic acid and treatment is by surgical excision.

Gastrointestinal Neurofibromas and Dysplastic Lesions

Gastrointestinal neurofibromas may present with pain, bleeding, or abdominal distension and dysplastic changes in the colon may produce constipation.[5,13]

Pregnancy

The commonest complication in pregnancy is a permanent increase in the number and size of cutaneous neurofibromas.[13] Blood pressure requires careful monitoring and women with pelvic neurofibromas may need a cesarean section if the neurofibroma is thought to pose a risk to normal delivery.

Genetic Diagnosis and Counseling

Prompt diagnosis of NF1 is important to ensure that patients and their families are counseled appropriately and monitored for disease complications. The majority of patients with NF1 can be diagnosed by careful history taking and clinical examination. Genetic testing may be useful in the situations described in Table 1.6 and patients with unusual phenotypes should be discussed with specialist neurofibromatosis centers.

Prenatal Testing

Genetic counseling is a prerequisite for people with NF1 who are considering having children. The risk of passing on the disease to a child is 1 in 2 and of having a severely affected infant is 1 in 12.[5,13] Prenatal testing is available but disease severity cannot be predicted with certainty.[13] Preimplantation genetic diagnosis is offered in some units for people with NF1, and avoids the need for therapeutic termination of pregnancy.[56] Genetic diagnosis is made on single cells that are extracted from a 3-day-old embryo and cells that are negative for NF1 are transferred to the mother.[56]

TABLE 1.6. Recommendations for considering *NF1* gene testing.

- Young children with six or more café au lait patches as the sole disease manifestation and no family history of NF1 – other features may not develop until early adulthood
- Children over 3 years old with 3–5 café au lait patches and no other NF1 manifestations
- People with unusual phenotypes – for example, abnormal pigment that can be confused with NF1 (see Chap. 3)
- Families with café au lait patches and freckling without neurofibromas who may have Legius syndrome and a good prognosis (see Chap. 3)

Genetic Counseling for Patients with Segmental NF1

People with segmental NF1 have a small but definite risk of transmitting generalized NF1 to an offspring and the risk is about 5%.[6,13] We have encountered a patient with unilateral groin freckling who subsequently had a child with generalized NF1. Some individuals with segmental NF1 find it very difficult to contemplate a 5% risk of having a child with generalized NF1 with the possibility of severe complications. These patients should be discussed with the specialist Complex NF1 centre in Manchester with a view to referral for counseling and for detection of the *NF1* gene mutation. This is done through a combination of RNA blood sampling (this method is more sensitive for finding low levels of a mosaic gene change) and if necessary by biopsy of the affected skin area is undertaken.[57]

Accuracy and Cost of NF1 Mutation Testing

Current techniques detect the disease causing mutation in 95% of people with NF1, but the gene is large and routine testing takes 3–4 weeks and reporting up to 8 weeks, at a cost of approximately £500–600.[58]

Assessment and Follow-up of People with NF1

Children (Table 1.7)

Children with complex disease complications should be referred to one of the specialist NF1 services. Community pediatricians are best placed to carry out at least annual assessments and follow-up of children with uncomplicated NF1. It is important for the clinician to maintain close links with the child's school and to facilitate yearly ophthalmology assessments, local speech and language support, and occupational therapy when necessary.

TABLE 1.7. Assessment of children with neurofibromatosis 1.

The following should be recorded at each annual visit:

- Development and progress at school
- Visual symptoms, visual acuity, color vision, and fundoscopy until age of 7 and then every 2 years until adulthood; visual fields at appropriate developmental age (optic pathway glioma, glaucoma)
- Height (abnormal pubertal development)
- Weight (abnormal pubertal development)
- Pubertal development (delayed/precocious puberty due to pituitary/hypothalamic lesions)
- Blood pressure (consider renal artery stenosis/pheochromocytoma)
- Cardiovascular examination (congenital heart disease especially pulmonary stenosis)
- Evaluation of spine (scoliosis and/or underlying plexiform neurofibroma
- Evaluation of skin (cutaneous, subcutaneous, and plexiform neurofibromas)
- System examination if specific symptoms

Source: Reproduced from Ferner et al.[13] With permission from BMJ publishing group 2011

Young People 16–25 Years

Young people aged 16–25 years require clinical and emotional support to cope with NF1, and common issues are the variability of the disease complications and the development of neurofibromas during adolescence. Young people should have an awareness of the inheritance pattern of NF1 and of timing and the opportunities for prenatal counseling. They may need advice about educational issues, applications for employment, and in tackling attitudes of their peer group toward NF1 (see Chap. 4).

Adults

People with complex NF1 require lifelong follow-up in a specialist NF1 service. Adults with uncomplicated NF1 do not always have access to dedicated neurofibromatosis clinics and it is important that they know when to ask for medical support for potentially serious problems. Annual blood pressure monitoring is essential, and people who develop symptomatic plexiform neurofibromas (see section on neurofibromas) or neurological problems suggestive of cord compression or tumor should seek urgent advice. Information and support may be obtained from the Neuro Foundation (formerly Neurofibromatosis Association) website and from the Foundation's specialist advisers who are based in different areas of the UK.

Nationally Commissioned "Complex NF1" Service (see Table 1.8)

NF1 is a complex condition with wide variation in clinical manifestations even in families. Many people have mild disease and cope very well with follow-up from general practitioners and local clinicians. However, some individuals suffer from rare complications that cause significant morbidity and may be life threatening. These individuals benefit from diagnosis, management and life-long surveillance, and support from specialist, multi-disciplinary NF1 teams who are conversant with rare clinical manifestations and linked nationally and internationally with other experts in the field. This permits optimum clinical and holistic care for patients and their families provided by consultant-led services that are abreast of the latest developments in therapy. Centralized care by a dedicated group of clinicians and nurses, improves the patient experience by coordinating care and reducing the need for multiple referrals to different specialists and hospitals. Specialist nurses act as patient advocates and as a link between the NF service and the community. The National Commissioning Group has funded Guy's and St. Thomas' NHS Foundation Trust as the lead center in England with Central Manchester Foundation Trust to care for patients with Complex NF1 and work with allied experts and local clinicians to provide the best possible management for this distressing disease (see also Chap. 4 and Appendix for contact details).

TABLE 1.8. NF1 complications that are managed by Nationally
Commissioned Complex NF1 Clinics.

- *Extensive symptomatic plexiform neurofibroma involving face,
  whole limb, pelvis, abdomen, or thorax*
  Role of NCG service: To discuss with experienced surgeon the
  need for surgery and to ensure the risks of hemorrhage, infection,
  neurological deficit, and recurrent tumor are understood by patient

- *MPNST*
  Role of NCG service: People with plexiform neurofibroma
  and persistent pain, rapid growth, hard texture, or unexplained
  neurological deficit require urgent referral and assessment in
  collaboration with specialist sarcoma units

- *Optic pathway glioma*
  Role of NCG service: Work with pediatric ophthalmologist/
  orthoptist to ensure annual visual screening for NF1 children;
  ensure MRI is not used for screening for OPG; and ensure children
  with known OPG are managed jointly by pediatric oncologist and
  pediatric ophthalmologists with experience in NF1

- *Cord compression from cervical plexiform neurofibroma*
  Role of NCG service: Ensure decisions regarding need for surgery
  are based on clinical findings as well as neuroimaging

- *Multiple sclerosis, aqueduct stenosis, brain glioma, and refractory
  epilepsy due to underlying structural lesion*
  Role of NCG service: Work with neurologists to ensure that the
  specific needs of the NF1 individual are taken into account when
  managing these complications

- *Pseudarthrosis of long bone*
  Role of NCG service: Education of pediatricians to avoid erroneous
  diagnosis of non-accidental injury. Ensure children are referred to
  orthopedic surgeons with specialist knowledge of this manifestation

- *Atypical phenotypes and counseling for segmental NF1*
  Role of NCG service: Ensure that people with unusual clinical
  presentations have appropriate clinical and genetic investigation
  to make the correct diagnosis. In rare instances, provide prenatal
  counseling and genetic testing for people with segmental NF1

References

1. Tilesius von Tilenau WG. *Historia pathologica singularis cutis turpitudinis. Jo Godfredi Rheinhardi viri Lannorum.* Leipzig, Germany: SL Crusius; 1793.
2. von Recklinghausen FD. *über die multiplen fibrome der haut und ihre beziehung zu den multiplen neuromen.* A Hirschwald, Berlin; 1882.
3. National Institutes of Health Consensus Development Conference Statement. Neurofibromatosis. *Arch Neurol Chicago.* 1988;45: 575-578.
4. Huson SM, Compston DAS, Clark P, et al. A genetic study of von Recklinghausen neurofibromatosis in south east Wales. 1. Prevalence, fitness, mutation rate, and effect of parental transmission on severity. *J Med Genet.* 1989;26:704-711.
5. Ferner RE. Neurofibromatosis 1 and neurofibromatosis 2: a twenty first century perspective. *Lancet Neurol.* 2007;6:340-351.
6. Ruggieri M, Huson SM. The clinical and diagnostic implications of mosaicism in the neurofibromatoses. *J Neurol.* 2001;56:1433-1443.
7. Viskochil D, Buchberg AN, Xu G, et al. Deletions and a translocation interrupt a cloned gene at the neurofibromatosis type 1 locus. *Cell.* 1990;62:1887-1892.
8. Wallace MR, Marchuk DA, Anderson LB, et al. Type 1 neurofibromatosis gene: identification of a larger transcript disrupted in three NG1 patients. *Science.* 1990;249:181-186.
9. Xu GF, O'Connell P, Viskochil D, et al. The neurofibromatosis type 1 gene encodes a protein related to GAP. *Cell.* 1990;62:599-608.
10. Johannessen CM, Reczek EE, James M, et al. The NF1 tumour suppressor critically regulates TSC2 and mTOR. *Proc Natl Acad Sci USA.* 2005;102:8573-8578.
11. Huson SM, Harper PS, Compston DAS. Von Recklinghausen neurofibromatosis: clinical and population study in south east Wales. *Brain.* 1988;111:55-81.
12. Brems H, Chmara M, Sahbatou M, et al. Germline loss of function mutations in SPRED1 cause a neurofibromatosis 1 – like phenotype. *Nat Genet.* 2007;39:1120-1126.
13. Ferner RE, Huson SM, Thomas N, et al. Guidelines for the diagnosis and management of individuals with neurofibromatosis 1. *J Med Genet.* 2007;44:81-88.
14. Cambiaghi S, Restano L, Caputo R. Juvenile xanthogranulomas associated with neurofibromatosis 1: 14 patients without evidence of haematologic malignancies. *Paediatr Dermatol.* 2004;21:97-101.
15. De Smet L, Sciot R, Legius E. Multifocal glomus tumours of the fingers in two patients with neurofibromatosis type 1. *J Med Genet.* 2002;39:e45.

16. Schindeler A, Little DG. Recent insights into bone development, homeostasis, and repair in type 1 neurofibromatosis (NF1). *Bone.* 2008;42:616-622.

17. Ferner RE. The neurofibromatoses. *Pract Neurol.* 2010;10:82-93.

18. Crawford AH Jr, Bagamery N. Osseous manifestations of neurofibromatosis in childhood. *J Pediatr Orthop.* 1986;6:72-88.

19. Cnossen MH, Moons KG, Garssen MP, et al. Minor disease features in neurofibromatosis type 1 (NF1) and their possible value in diagnosis of NF1 in children < or =6 years and clinically suspected of having NF1. Neurofibromatosis team of Sophia Children's Hospital. *J Med Genet.* 1998;35:624-627.

20. Tucker T, Schnabel C, Hartmann M, et al. Bone health and fracture rate in individuals with neurofibromatosis 1 (NF1). *J Med Genet.* 2009;46:259-265.

21. Howlett DC, Farrugia MM, Ferner RE, et al. Multiple lower limb non-ossifying neurofibromas in siblings with neurofibromatosis. *Eur J Radiol.* 1998;26:280-283.

22. Casselman ES, Mandell GA. Vertebral scalloping in neurofibromatosis. *Radiology.* 1979;131:89-94.

23. Kimura M, Kamata Y, Matsumoto K, et al. Electron microscopical study on the tumour of von Recklinghausen's neurofibromatosis. *Acta Pathol Jpn.* 1974;24:79-91.

24. Lammert M, Mautner VF, Kluwe L. Do hormonal contraceptives stimulate growth of neurofibromas? A survey on 59 NF1 patients. *BMC Cancer.* 2005;5:16.

25. Evans DGR, Huson S, Donnai D, et al. A clinical study of type 2 neurofibromatosis. *Q J Med.* 1992;84:603-618.

26. MacCollin M, Chiocca EA, Evans DG, et al. Diagnostic criteria for Schwannomatosis. *Neurology.* 2005;64:1838-1845.

27. Sharif S, Moran A, Huson SM, et al. Women with neurofibromatosis 1 are at a moderately increased risk of developing breast cancer and should be considered for early screening. *J Med Genet.* 2007;44: 481-484.

28. Leonard JR, Ferner RE, Thomas N, et al. Cervical cord compression from plexiform neurofibromas in neurofibromatosis 1. *J Neurol Neurosurg Psychiatry.* 2007;78:1404-1406.

29. Mautner VF, Asuagbor FA, Dombi E, et al. Assessment of benign tumour burden by whole-body MRI in patients with neurofibromatosis 1. *Neuro Oncol.* 2008;10:593-598.

30. Evans DG, Baser ME, McGraughran J, et al. Malignant peripheral nerve sheath tumours in neurofibromatosis 1. *J Med Genet.* 2002;39:311-314.

31. Ferner RE, Gutmann D. International Consensus Group Statement of the management of malignant peripheral nerve sheath tumours in neurofibromatosis 1. *Cancer Res.* 2002;62:1573-1577.

32. Ferner RE, Golding JF, Smith M, et al. [18F] 2-fluoro-2-deoxy-D-glucose positron emission tomography (FDG PET) as a diagnostic

tool for neurofibromatosis 1 (NF1) associated malignant peripheral nerve sheath tumours (MPNSTs): a long-term clinical study. *Ann Oncol.* 2008;19:390-394.

33. Ferner RE, Hughes RA, Hall SM, et al. Neurofibromatous neuropathy in neurofibromatosis 1 (NF1). *J Med Genet.* 2004;41:837-841.

34. North K, Riccardi V, Samango-Sprouse C, et al. Cognitive function and academic performance in NF1: consensus statement from the NF1 cognitive disorders task force. *Neurology.* 1997;48:1121-1127.

35. Costa RM, Silva AJ. Molecular and cellular mechanisms underlying the cognitive deficits associated with neurofibromatosis 1. *J Child Neurol.* 2002;17:622-626.

36. Krab LC, de Goede-Bolder A, Aarsen FK, et al. Effect of simvastatin on cognitive functioning in children with neurofibromatosis type 1: a randomised controlled trial. *JAMA.* 2008;300:287-294.

37. Créange A, Zeller J, Rostaing-Rigattieri S, et al. Neurological complications of neurofibromatosis type 1 in adulthood. *Brain.* 1999;122:473-481.

38. Gill DS, Hyman SL, Steinberg A, North KN. Age-related findings on MRI in neurofibromatosis type 1. *Pediatr Radiol.* 2006;36:1048-1056.

39. Hyman SL, Gill DS, Shores EA, et al. T2 hyperintensities in children with neurofibromatosis type 1 and their relationship to cognitive functioning. *J Neurol Neurosurg Psychiatry.* 2007;78:1088-1091.

40. Listernick R, Ferner RE, Liu GT, et al. Optic pathway gliomas in neurofibromatosis-1: controversies and recommendations. *Ann Neurol.* 2007;61:189-198.

41. Listernick R, Ferner RE, Piersall L, et al. Late-onset optic pathway tumours in children with neurofibromatosis 1. *Neurology.* 2004;63:194-196.

42. Sharif S, Ferner R, Birch JM, et al. Second primary tumours in neurofibromatosis 1 patients treated for optic glioma: substantial risks after radiotherapy. *J Clin Oncol.* 2006;24:2570-2575.

43. Packer RJ, Alter J, Allen J, et al. Carboplatin and vincristine chemotherapy for children with newly diagnosed progressive low-grade gliomas. *J Neurosurg.* 1997;86:747-754.

44. Dasgupta B, Yi Y, Chen DY, et al. Proteomic analysis reveals hyperactivation of the mammalian target of rapacmycin pathway in neurofibromatosis 1-associated human and mouse brain tumours. *Cancer Res.* 2005;1:2755-2760.

45. Schonauer C, Tessitore E, Frascadore L, et al. Lumbosacral dural ectasia in type 1 neurofibromatosis. Report of two cases. *Neurosurg Sci.* 2000;44:165-168.

46. Vivarelli R, Grosso S, Calabrese F. Epilepsy in neurofibromatosis 1. *J Child Neurol.* 2003;18:338-342.

47. Johnson MR, Ferner RE, Bobrow M, et al. Detailed analysis of the oligodendrocyte myelin glycoprotein gene in four patients with neurofibromatosis 1 and primary progressive multiple sclerosis. *J Neurol Neurosurg Psychiatry.* 2000;8:643-646.

48. Rea D, Brandsema JF, Armstrong D. Cerebral arteriopathy in children with neurofibromatosis type 1. *Pediatrics*. 2009;124:e476-e483.
49. Rosser TL, Vezina G, Packer RT. Cerebrovascular abnormalities in a population of children with neurofibromatosis type 1. *Neurology*. 2005;64:553-555.
50. Friedman JM, Arbiser J, Epstein JA, et al. Cardiovascular disease in neurofibromatosis 1: a report of the NF1 Cardiovascular Task Force. *Genet Med*. 2003;4:105-111.
51. Lisch K. Ueber beteiligung der augen, insbesondere das vorkommen von irisknotchen bei der neurofibromatose (Recklinghausen). *Z Augenheilkunde*. 1937;93:137-143.
52. Srinivasan A, Krishnamurthy G, Fontalvo-Herazo L, et al. Spectrum of renal findings in paediatric fibromuscular dysplasia and neurofibromatosis type 1. *Pediatr Radiol*. 2010 Oct 16. Epub ahead of print.
53. Bausch B, Borozdin W, Neumann H, et al. Clinical and genetic characteristics of patients with neurofibromatosis type 1 and phaeochromocytoma. *NEJM*. 2006;354:2729-2731.
54. Miettinen M, Fetsch JF, Sobin LH, et al. Gastrointestinal stromal tumours in patients with neurofibromatosis 1: a clinicopathologic and molecular genetic study of 45 cases. *Am J Surg Pathol*. 2006;30:90-96.
55. Hough DR, Usar MC, Chan A, et al. Von Recklinghausen's disease associated with gastrointestinal carcinoid tumours. *Cancer*. 1983;51:2206-2208.
56. Verlinsky Y, Rechitsky S, Verlinsky O, et al. Preimplantation diagnosis for neurofibromatosis. *Reprod Biomed Online*. 2002;4:218-222.
57. Maertens O, De Schepper S, Vandesompele J, et al. Molecular dissection of isolated disease features in mosaic neurofibromatosis type 1. *Am J Hum Genet*. 2007;81:243-251.
58. Upadhyaya M. Neurofibromatosis type 1: diagnosis and recent advances. *Expert Opin Med Diagn*. 2010;4:307-322.

Chapter 2
Neurofibromatosis Type 2 (NF2)

D. Gareth R. Evans

Terminology

Disease Name and Synonyms

Neurofibromatosis type 2 (NF2), Bilateral acoustic neurofibromatosis, Central neurofibromatosis. OMIM #101000. The correct name for the condition is Neurofibromatosis type 2 (NF2). The remaining names are historically due to the overlap with NF1 and previous confusion over the two conditions. The first clear description of NF2 was in 1822 by Wishart.[1] NF1 was described in 1882 by von Recklinghausen. However, it was Harvey Cushing who described bilateral eighth nerve tumors developing as part of von Recklinghausen disease in 1916.[2] This description is largely responsible for the confusion between the two conditions which continued for many years. Gradually over the last 20 years of the twentieth century the clear clinical and pathological differences resulted in the definition of two separate conditions, NF1, formerly known as von Recklinghausen neurofibromatosis and NF2 previously called bilateral acoustic or central neurofibromatosis. The clinical and genetic distinction between the two conditions was not fully recognized until the last three decades and reports of "neurofibromatosis" frequently included intermingled NF1 and NF2 cases.[3] The conditions were eventually recognized as

R.E. Ferner et al., *Neurofibromatoses in Clinical Practice*,
DOI: 10.1007/978-0-85729-629-0_2,
© Springer-Verlag London Limited 2011

separate entities with the localization of the respective genes to chromosome 17 and 22.[4,5] This was followed by the formal clinical delineation at a US National Institutes of Health (NIH) consensus meeting in 1987.[6]

Diagnosis

The Manchester (modified NIH) diagnostic criteria for NF2 are shown in Table 2.1. The original NIH criteria[6] have been expanded to include patients with no family history who have multiple schwannomas and or meningiomas, but who have not yet developed bilateral 8th nerve tumors.[7] The diagnosis is best confirmed using high quality MRI imaging of the brain (with 3 mm cuts through the internal auditory meati) with gadolinium enhancement. Full spinal axis imaging should also be performed. Examination of the skin for NF2 intracutaneous and deeper subcutaneous nodules is useful although, where the diagnosis is in doubt and depends on verification of a cutaneous tumor, biopsy should be considered. Ophthalmic examination with a slit lamp is also advised. *NF2* is the only gene known to be associated with neurofibromatosis 2. Molecular genetic testing of *NF2* that includes a combination of sequence analysis or mutation scanning and

TABLE 2.1. Diagnostic criteria for NF2 (these include the NIH criteria with additional criteria).

Bilateral vestibular schwannomas *or* family history of NF2 *plus*
1. Unilateral VS *or* 2. Any two of: meningioma, glioma, neurofibroma, schwannoma, posterior subcapsular lenticular opacities
Additional criteria: Unilateral VS *plus* any two of: meningioma, glioma, neurofibroma, schwannoma, and posterior subcapsular opacities
Or
Multiple meningioma (two or more) *plus* unilateral VS *or* any two of: glioma, neurofibroma, schwannoma, and cataract

duplication/deletion testing detects a mutation in most affected individuals who have a positive family history and are not the first individual in the family known to have the disorder. Identification of a pathogenic *NF2* mutation in blood or in two anatomically distinct tumors from the same individual confirms the diagnosis.

Epidemiology

NF2 is an autosomal dominant disease that usually has a 50% risk of transmission from an affected individual to their off-spring. This was first confirmed in a large family reported by Gardner and Frazier in 1930. Fifty to sixty percent of patients have no family history and represent de novo mutations in the *NF2* gene.[7-10] Individuals who inherit a pathogenic mutation in the *NF2* gene will almost always develop symptoms by 60 years of age.[7] There have only been two epidemiological studies of NF2, one in North West England[8-10] and one in Finland.[11] The birth incidence of NF2 is most probably around 1:33,000 individuals,[10] with disease prevalence around 1 in 60,000.[10] Although the transmission rate is 50% in the second generation and beyond, the risk of transmission in an apparently isolated patient with NF2 is less than 50% due to mosaicism.[12]

Mosaicism

This is a phenomenon whereby the *NF2* mutation is only present in some of the affected individual's cells. A consider-able proportion of NF2 patients, particularly milder cases, have mosaic disease, in which only a proportion of cells con-tain the mutated *NF2* gene. The initiating mutation occurs after conception, leading to two separate cell lineages. The proportion of cells affected depends on how early in develop-ment the mutation occurs. Recent evidence suggests that between 20% and 33% of NF2 cases without a family history of the disease are mosaic, mostly carrying the mutation in too small a proportion or none of their lymphocytes to be detected from a blood sample.[12-15] This accounts for the milder disease course in many individuals with unfound mutations, and since only a subset of germ cells (or none) will carry the mutation, there is less than a 50% risk of transmitting the disease to their offspring. However, if an offspring has inherited the mutation, they will have a typical phenotype and usually be more severely affected than their parent, since the offspring will carry the mutation in all of their cells. The mosaic mutation can be detected by analyzing tumor material from an affected individual. If an identical mutation is found in two tumors from that individual, this confirms that this is the underlying mosaic mutation even if it cannot be identified in lymphocyte DNA. Their offspring can be tested for the presence of the mutation to exclude NF2. Offspring can also be tested for NF2 if both abnormalities are identified in a single tumor to also potentially exclude the disease. The chances of mosaicism based on different ages at presentation and whether NF2 presents symmetrically is shown in Table 2.2.

Clinical Manifestations

The hallmark of NF2 is the development of bilateral vestibular schwannomas (VS) (Figs. 2.1 and 2.2). The other main tumor features are schwannomas of the other cranial, spinal (Fig. 2.3) and peripheral nerves; meningiomas both intracranial (Figs. 2.1 and 2.4) also including optic nerve and intraspinal meningiomas and intraspinal; and some low-grade central nervous system (CNS) malignancies (ependymomas). Four large clinical studies have now confirmed this clinical picture.[7,16-18] Although the disease is still classified as "neurofibromatosis," neurofibromas are relatively infrequent. Individuals may present with cranial meningiomas or a spinal tumor long before the appearance of a VS.[19] Previously, there was a suggestion for two forms of the disease.[17,18] The Wishart type is more aggressive with an onset commonly in the late teens or with multi tumor disease, whereas the Gardner type

TABLE 2.2.   Chances of mosaicism and risk to offspring based on testing 402 de novo NF2 patients fulfilling Manchester Criteria.

Diagnosis of VS[a]	Number of patients	Mutation non-mosaic	Mosaic found blood	Mosaic found tumor	Mosaic inferred pre blood genetic test (%)	Transmission risk pre blood genetic test (%)	Likelihood of a missed full mutation after negative blood testing	Mosaic inferred post negative blood testing (%)	Transmission risk post negative blood testing
<20 BVS	99	81 (81%)	5 (5%)	1 (1%)	12	45	7/13 (54%)	46	29% 1 in 3
<20 UVS	21	13 (62%)	3 (14%)	3 (14%)	33	33	1.1/5 (22%)	78	15% 1 in 7
20–29 BVS	77	49 (64%)	7 (9%)	2 (3%)	30	36	4.3/21 (20%)	80	15% 1 in 7
20–29 UVS	28	5 (18%)	4 (14%)	6 (21%)	78	19	0.44/19 (2%)	98	6% 1 in 16
30–39 BVS	54	25 (45%)	9 (17%)	7 (13%)	50	28	2.2/20 (11%)	89	11% 1 in 9
30–39 UVS	20	3 (15%)	1 (5%)	6 (30%)	83	12	0.26/16 (2%)	98	6% 1 in 16
40+ BVS	59	18 (31%)	5 (8%)	7 (12%)	66	22	1.56/26 (6%)	94	9% 1 in 11
40+ UVS	44	4 (9%)	2 (5%)	8 (18%)	90	10	0.35/36 (1%)	99	5.5% 1 in 20
Total	402	198 (49%)	36 (9%)	40 (10%)					

[a] Age at diagnosis of VS in patients fulfilling at least Manchester criteria

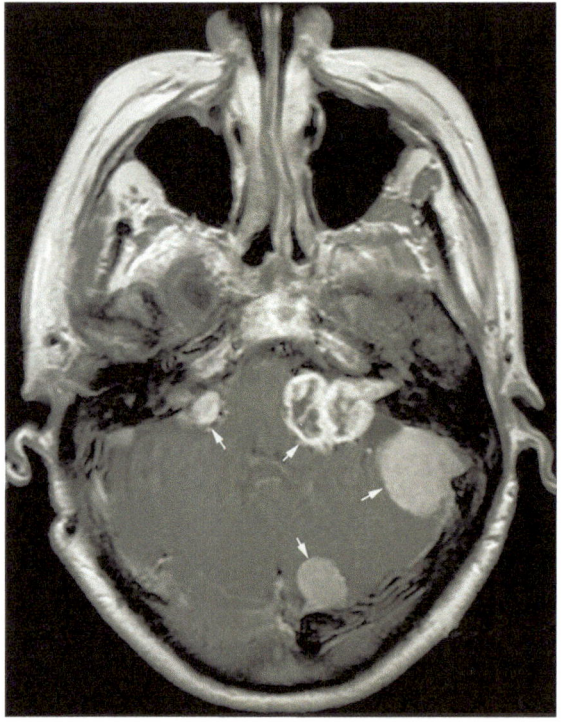

FIGURE 2.1. Cranial MRI showing bilateral vestibular schwannomas and meningiomas.

usually presents in an older age group with fewer tumors and perhaps only bilateral VS. In practice, classification into Gardner and Wishart type is often difficult and may vary between family members. In reality, the variation is a combination of chance, other risk factors, other genes, and the *NF2* mutation type.

In the same way as sporadic VS, the majority of adults with NF2 present with hearing loss that is usually unilateral at time of onset. Nausea, vomiting, or true vertigo are rare symptoms except in late stage disease. A significant proportion of cases (20–30%) present with symptoms from an intracranial meningioma (headaches, seizures), spinal tumor (pain, muscle weakness, paresthesia), or cutaneous tumor.[7,16-]

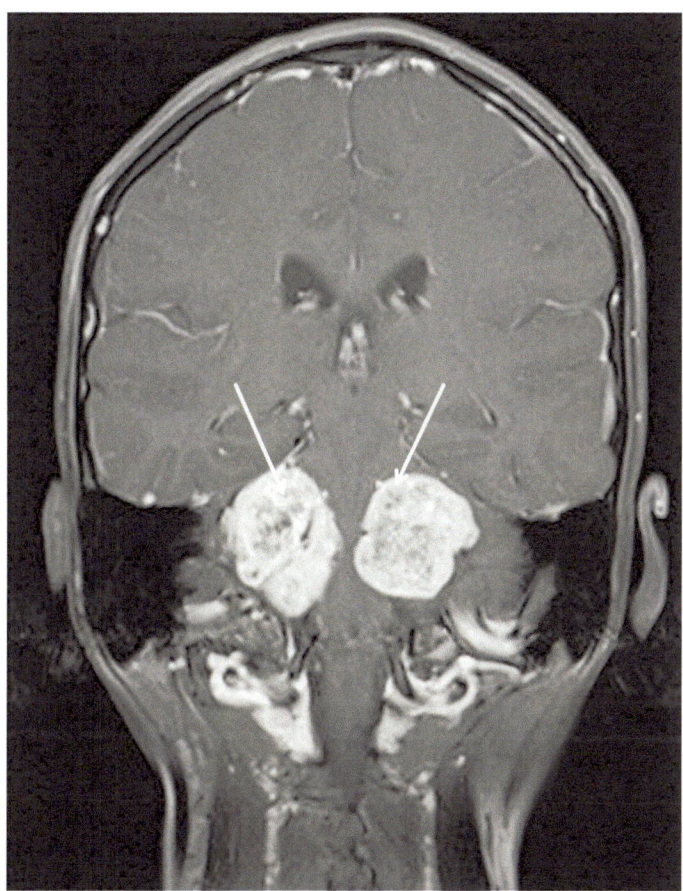

FIGURE 2.2. Bilateral massive vestibular schwannomas compressing the brain stem.

[18] Indeed, the first sign of more severe multi-tumor disease in early childhood is often a non-eighth nerve tumor (including a cutaneous tumor), an ocular presentation, or a mononeuropathy, which frequently affects the facial nerve.[19,20] Some children present with a polio-like illness with wasting of muscle groups in a lower limb (amyotrophy), which usually does not fully recover. In adulthood, a more generalized symptomatic severe polyneuropathy occurs in about 3–10%

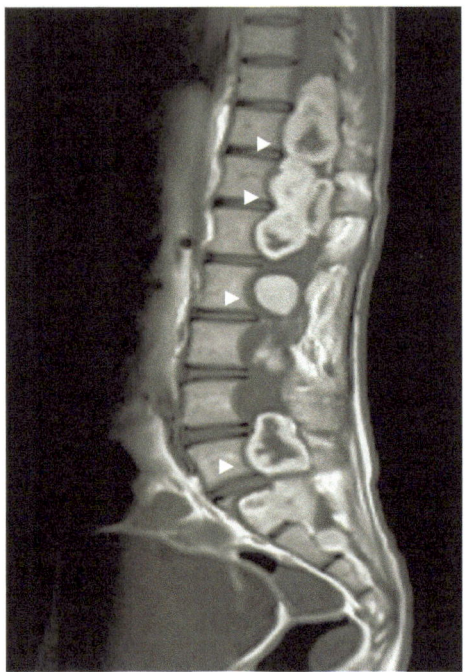

FIGURE 2.3. Multiple spinal schwannomas some with cystic change in NF2 as indicated by *arrows*.

of patients, often associated with an "onion bulb" appearance on nerve biopsy.[7] Around 40% of patients will show evidence of polyneuropathy on nerve conduction studies.[21]

Ophthalmic features are also prominent in NF2. Patients often suffer from reduced visual acuity of various causes. Many of these are amblyopias with no obvious cause. Between 60% and 80% of patients have cataracts and these may present in early life.[7,16,17] These can be posterior subcapsular lenticular opacities or cortical wedge opacities. Optic nerve meningiomas can cause visual loss in the first years of life and extensive retinal hamartomas can also affect vision.

The skin is a useful aid to diagnosis, but cutaneous features in NF2 are much more subtle than in NF1. About 70% of

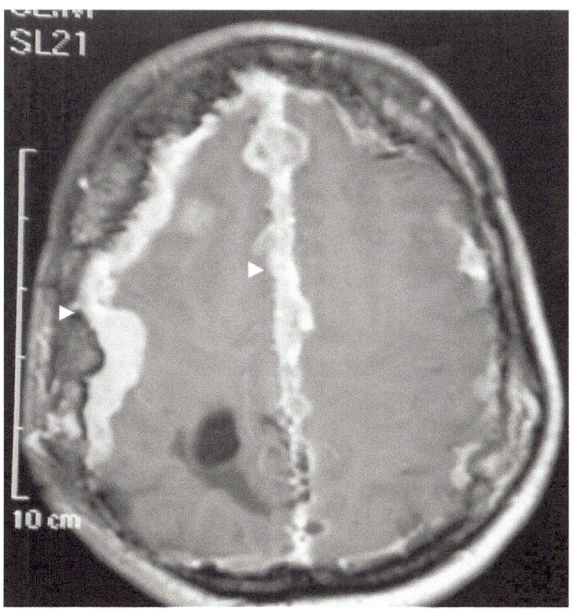

FIGURE 2.4. En plaque meningioma affecting most of the meninges including the falx.

NF2 patients have skin-related tumors, but only 10% have more than ten skin tumors.[7] The most frequent type is a plaque-like lesion, which is intracutaneous, slightly raised and more pigmented than surrounding skin, often with excess hair (Fig. 2.5). More deep-seated subcutaneous nodular tumors can often be felt, sometimes on major peripheral nerves (Fig. 2.6). Café au lait patches are more frequent in NF2 than in the general population but are rarely as frequent as in NF1 with only 1% having six or more patches.[7]

Screening At-Risk Individuals

Children of affected patients should be considered to be at 50% risk of NF2 and screening for NF2 can start at birth with a search for cataracts. Formal screening for VS should start at

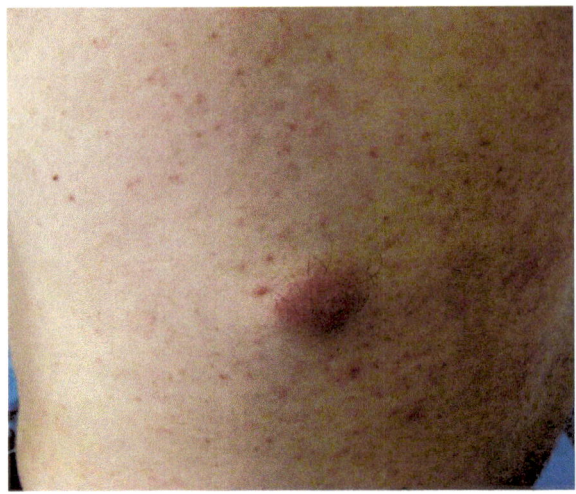

FIGURE 2.5. NF2 intracutaneous plaque: slightly raised, often pigmented with excess hair.

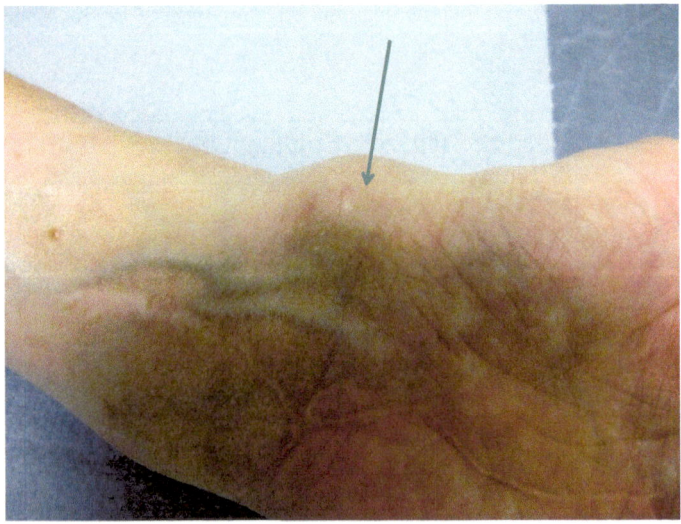

FIGURE 2.6. Ulnar nerve nodular subcutaneous schwannoma separate from overlying skin.

10 years, as it is rare for tumors to become symptomatic before that time even in severely affected families. Magnetic resonance imaging (MRI) of the head and spine is the mainstay of current screening, although annual audiological tests including auditory brainstem response are still a useful adjunct to MRI.[22] VS growth is faster in younger patients, so for asymptomatic at-risk individuals without tumors, MRI screening every 2 years for those younger than 20 years old is recommended. For those older than 20 years MRI screening every 3–5 years should be sufficient. The initial MRI scan could be at around 12 years of age, or 10 years of age in severely affected families.

In most families, it is now possible to develop a genetic test so that screening can be targeted to affected individuals only. Identifying the affected patient's mutation not only allows testing of at-risk relatives, but may also give important indicators as to the patient's own prognosis. As 20–33% of de novo NF2 patients are mosaic, frozen tumor should be taken at operation (with patient consent) for genetic tests. Once a mutation is known in a family, testing for the specific mutation takes 2–3 weeks. Finding the family mutation on initial search usually takes 8–10 weeks and may take longer if tumor tests need to be performed. In the occasional family, with more than one affected family member in which a mutation cannot be found, linkage tests can still be used.

Surveillance

Once tumors are present or a mutation has been found in an affected child, MRI screening should probably be at least annual. Spinal tumors are seen in 60–80% of NF2 patients on MRI.[23] Nonetheless, only 25–30% of patients with spinal tumors require a spinal operation from a symptomatic tumor. Spinal MRI only every 3 years is probably sufficient unless there are new symptoms.[24] If no tumors are present on the initial scan, a further scan 5–10 years later may be reasonable.

Managing Affected Children

NF2 is being recognized more and more frequently in childhood often before VS have developed. Recognition of the more severe disease course with early presentation and the more atypical features such as mononeuropathy are important.

Screening Individuals with Insufficient Criteria for NF2

Many individuals have two NF2-related tumors or present at very young ages with VS or meningioma, and are clearly at risk of at least having mosaic NF2. Twenty percent of patients <20 years with a sporadic VS will develop NF2[25] but only half of these will have a detectable mutation on blood DNA. Similarly, around 20% of apparently sporadic childhood meningioma develops into NF2.[20] Individuals who present with a unilateral VS and other neurogenic tumors in the NF2 spectrum have a high risk of contralateral disease especially if they present at age <20 years.[26] Five yearly MRI should probably be performed at least until 40 years of age in individuals with a sporadic VS <30 years or a meningioma <20 years of age.

Genetics

NF1 and NF2 were eventually recognized as separate genetic and clinical diseases with the localization of the respective genes to chromosome 17 and 22.[27,28] This was followed by the formal clinical delineation at a National Institutes of Health (NIH) consensus meeting in the USA, in 1987.[6]

The *NF2* gene was isolated by the simultaneous discovery of constitutional and tumor deletions in a gene coding for a cell membrane-related protein, which has been termed merlin or schwannomin by the two groups who isolated it.[4,5] This protein is involved in the interaction between actin within the cell cytoskeleton and the cell membrane, and appears to suppress tumorigenesis through contact-mediated growth inhibition.

The majority of mutations in the *NF2* gene are truncating mutations, leading to a smaller and probably nonfunctional protein product. Early studies suggested that missense mutations (which result in a complete protein product) and large deletions (which result in no protein product) both cause mild phenotypes. Larger studies of detailed genotype/phenotype correlations in multiple families have confirmed this finding.[29-36] The phenotype is more variable in patients with splice-site mutations, with milder disease in patients with mutations in exons 9–15.[32,35] This variation in disease severity is reflected in longer survival for those patients with a missense mutation compared to those with a truncating mutation.[34] Large scale genomic rearrangements may also occur and account for around 15% of NF2 germline aberrations.[37,38]

The sensitivity of genetic testing using sequence analysis and MLPA is around 92% as this is the detection rate in the second generation of NF2 families.[13]

Differential Diagnosis

The main differential diagnosis of NF2 is schwannomatosis (Table 2.3[39]) however some patients with multiple non-cranial schwannomas turn out to have mosaic NF2.[40,41] However one exclusion criteria of schwannomatosis is vestibular schwannoma, it is still not entirely clear that these do not occur in schwannomatosis. Final confirmation of schwannomatosis would involve confirming different *NF2* mutations in schwannomas from the same individual or identification of a *SMARCB1* mutation.[42] Patients fulfilling the most sensitive Manchester criteria are unlikely to be misclassified.[43] Care must be taken to be sure that bilateral enhancing lesions in the Cerebellopontine angle are vestibular schwannoma. These can be due to metastatic processes from choroid plexus carcinoma, lymphoma, ependymoma, or melanoma.

TABLE 2.3. Diagnostic criteria for schwannomatosis.

Definite	Possible
Age *over* 30 years AND two or more non-intradermal schwannomas, at least 1 with histologic confirmation AND no evidence of vestibular tumor on high-quality MRI scan AND no known constitutional *NF2* mutation	Age *under* 30 years AND two or more non-intradermal schwannomas, at least 1 with histologic confirmation AND no evidence of vestibular tumor on high quality MRI scan AND no known constitutional *NF2* mutation
Or	*Or*
One pathologically confirmed schwannoma plus a first-degree relative who meets above criteria	Age over 45 years AND two or more non-intradermal schwannomas, at least one with histologic confirmation AND no symptoms of 8th nerve dysfunction AND no known constitutional *NF2* mutation
	Or
	Radiographic evidence of a schwannoma and first degree relative meeting criteria for definite schwannomatosis

Segmental

Meets criteria for either definite or possible schwannomatosis but limited to one limb or five or fewer contiguous segments of the spine

NF2 Management

Surgery

VS surgery in NF2 presents unique technical and decision-making challenges. Schwannomas in the cerebellopontine angle may have multifocal components from the eighth nerve as well as from adjacent cranial nerves – facial, trigeminal, and the lower cranial nerves. As a result, the facial nerve may pass though the middle of the tumor mass and be difficult to identify. The principle of surgery is to limit the burden of neurological deficit as far as is possible. Facial nerve preservation is very important in the presence of bilateral disease. Facial paralysis threatens the health of the eye by loss of blink and lacrimation (loss of intermedius nerve function), and if combined with trigeminal damage is a serious threat to vision. Risk is minimized by leaving fragments of VS on the facial nerve and if possible by not removing a coexistent facial schwannoma. The patient should be considered holistically. If the vision on the contralateral side is poor (not an infrequent finding in NF2), then surgery should be very conservative. Similar arguments apply to the management of the lower cranial nerves to avoid the problems of bilateral bulbar palsy. "Do not remove a tumor just because it is there!" Usually a VS with good hearing will be treated conservatively until there is a neurosurgical need to remove it. However, there are occasions, when early removal of small tumors will be advised if it is felt possible to preserve hearing or at worst the cochlear nerve for subsequent cochlear implantation. Surgical results are certainly far better when managed by an experienced team.[24,44-47] There is clear evidence of a reduction in mortality with a significantly increased life expectancy for NF2 patients managed at three specialty centers in the UK (OR 0.34).[47] All other craniospinal axis tumors should also be managed conservatively with a goal of preserving function. The removal of asymptomatic tumors should only be undertaken if there is evidence of rapid growth and inevitable loss of function without surgery.[24] All NF2 patients should be managed in the context of a multidisciplinary team with a minimum of an NF2 physician, ENT surgeon, Neurosurgeon, and neuroradiologist.[24]

Radiotherapy

The use of radiotherapy is controversial in patients with NF2 although it may be useful in some situations. The same tumor considerations make treatment results worse in NF2 than in sporadic disease.[48] It has a role in patients who have particularly aggressive tumors, who are poor surgical candidates or who refuse surgery. This should be weighed against control rates of only 50% compared to a control rate in sporadic VS of 95%.[48,49] In addition, there is a greater risk of malignant change in NF2 patients compared to sporadic VS.[50,51] Forty percent of patients retain pretreatment hearing for at least 3 years. The upper limit of size for radiotherapy is generally a maximum intracranial diameter of 3 cm.[48] It is important to be able to offer both radiotherapy and surgery, and both options should be discussed in a balanced fashion. Surgeons should use clinical judgment as to when to recommend radiation therapy.[24,48]

Hearing Rehabilitation

Hearing preservation surgery in patients with NF2 is extremely difficult. Patients often become bilaterally profoundly deaf as a result of the disease or treatment of the disease. Teams experienced in the positioning of brainstem implants can offer partial auditory rehabilitation to those who are deaf, although results are still behind those achievable for cochlear implants. In a few patients, it may be possible to rehabilitate hearing successfully with a cochlear implant if the cochlear nerve is left intact after surgery. However, this is not always possible even in the presence of an intact nerve as its blood supply may be damaged. The Auditory Brainstem Implant (ABI, Cochlear Nucleus Implant) has allowed most recipients to appreciate environmental noise and to enhance their lip reading skills. A small number are able to achieve good open set sentence scores, but as yet the factors that predict outcome are not fully understood.

New Therapies

The NF2 protein appears to impact on multiple intracellular signaling pathways. These pathways include the PI3-kinase, mTOR, Akt, and Raf/MEK/ERK pathways.[52]

The progress being made in cellular research especially with regard to pathways in which the NF2 gene product interacts raises the hopes of targeted therapy. Targeting the ERK1/, AKT, integrin/focal adhesion kinase/Src/Ras signaling cascades, PDGFRbeta, phosphatidylinositol 3-kinase/protein kinase C/Src/c-Raf pathway, VEG-F, and other pathways[52] means that drugs such as bevacizumab, erlotinib, lapatinib, and sorafenib[53] may well bear fruit. Indeed, a recent report on ten patients showed objective radiological improvement in eight VS with bevacizumab.[54] A further small report on two German patients treated with bevacizumab backs up the promise of drug treatments.[55]

Genetic Counseling and Prenatal Counseling

Mode of Inheritance

Neurofibromatosis 2 (NF2) is inherited in an autosomal dominant manner.

Risk to Family Members

Parents of a Proband

Around 50% of individuals with NF2 have an affected parent, and 50% have NF2 as the result of a de novo mutation. However, 25–33% of individuals who are simplex cases (i.e., individuals with no family history of NF2) are mosaic for an *NF2* mutation.[13,14]

Recommendations for the evaluation of parents of a proband with an apparent de novo mutation include a clinical history and, if any suspicion of NF2 exists, an MRI scan. A parent can be excluded as having NF2 if his/her offspring is shown to be mosaic, but absence of a mutation detected in the child does not eliminate the possibility of mosaicism in the parent. Because the age of onset of symptoms is consistent within families, it is usually not necessary to offer surveillance to asymptomatic parents.

Sibs of a Proband

The risk to the sibs of the proband depends on the genetic status of the parents.

- If a parent of the proband is affected, the risk to the sibs is 50%.
- If neither parent of an individual with NF2 is symptomatic, the risk to the sibs of the affected individual is extremely low because the age of onset of symptoms is relatively uniform within families.
- However, a single case of germline mosaicism in a clinically normal individual has been reported.[17]

Offspring of a Proband

Each child of an individual with NF2 has up to a 50% chance of inheriting the mutation:

- If the proband has other affected family members, each child of the proband has a 50% chance of inheriting the mutation.
- If the proband is the only affected individual in the family, two possibilities exist:
  - The proband may have somatic mosaicism for the disease-causing mutation. Offspring of an individual who is mosaic will have less than a 50% risk chance of inheriting the disease-causing mutation. The proband may have a de novo germline mutation (i.e., present in the egg or sperm at the time of conception). Each offspring of an individual with a de novo germline mutation has a 50% chance of inheriting the mutation.
- Persons with somatic mosaicism and bilateral vestibular schwannomas have <50% chance of having an affected child. If a point mutation is detected in DNA from multiple tumors, but not in DNA from leukocytes, the risk to offspring is probably less than 5%.[13]

Other Family Members of a Proband

The risk to other family members depends on the genetic status of the proband's parents. If a parent is found to be affected, his or her family members may be at risk, depending on the family structure.

Predictive Testing

At-risk relatives whose genetic status is unknown can be tested for presence of the *NF2* mutation (either constitutional or somatic mosaic) identified in an affected relative such as the proband. In the rare instance in which an *NF2* mutation cannot be identified, linkage analysis can be used in families with at least two affected family members of different generations or tumor DNA can be used to exclude at least half of children as being at risk.

Offspring of a sporadic case in whom molecular genetic testing of a tumor has revealed loss of heterozygosity (LOH) can be reassured if testing of their lymphocyte DNA shows that they have inherited the allele that was lost in the parental tumor, because this allele is unlikely to have a disease-causing mutation.[13,14]

Prenatal diagnosis/preimplantation genetic diagnosis (PGD) for at-risk pregnancies requires prior identification of the disease-causing mutation in the family. There is a limited but clear demand for this in some families.

Complications That Require Referral to National NF Centers

All NF2 patients should be managed under the auspices of a national center. Auditory brain stem implantation should only be carried out by an experienced team within a national center. Some especially milder cases of NF2 can have their main management carried out by a multidrug therapy (MDT) in a peripheral center with regional review annually by the Regional MDT.

Conclusions

NF2 continues to be a condition with considerable morbidity and increased mortality. Multidisciplinary management with early diagnosis is vital for management. Hopefully, new targeted therapies will revolutionize the outcomes in this condition.

References

1. Wishart JH. Case of tumours in the skull, dura mater, and brain. *Edinburgh Med Surg J*. 1822;18:393-397.
2. Cushing H. *Tumours of the Nervus Acusticus and the Syndrome of the Cerebello-pontine Angle*. Philadelphia: WB Saunders; 1917.
3. Crowe FW, Schull WJ, Neal JV, eds. *A Clinical Pathological and Genetic Study of Multiple Neurofibromatosis*. Springfield, IL: Charles C. Thomas; 1956.
4. Rouleau GA, Merel P, Lutchman M, et al. Alteration in a new gene encoding a putative membrane-organizing protein causes neuro-fibromatosis type 2. *Nature*. 1993;363:515-521.
5. Troffater JA, MacCollin MM, Rutter JL, et al. A novel moesin-, ezrin-, radixin-like gene is a candidate for the neurofibromatosis 2 tumour suppressor. *Cell*. 1993;72:791-800.
6. National Institutes of Health Consensus Development Conference. Statement on neurofibromatosis. *Arch Neurol*. 1987;45:575-579.
7. Evans DGR, Huson S, Donnai D, et al. A clinical study of type 2 neurofibromatosis. *Q J Med*. 1992;84:603-618.
8. Evans DGR, Huson SM, Donnai D, et al. A genetic study of type 2 neurofibromatosis in the north west of England and the UK: I. Prevalence, mutation rate, fitness and confirmation of maternal transmission effect on severity. *J Med Genet*. 1992;29:841-846.

9. Evans DGR, Moran A, King A, Saeed S, Gurusinghe N, Ramsden R. Incidence of vestibular schwannoma and neurofibromatosis 2 in the North West of England over a 10 year period: higher incidence than previously thought. *Otol Neurotol*. 2005;26(1):93-97.

10. Evans DG, Howard E, Giblin C, et al. Birth incidence and prevalence of tumour prone syndromes: estimates from a UK genetic family register service. *Am J Med Genet*. 2010;152A(2):327-332.

11. Antinheimo J, Sankila R, Carpén O, Pukkala E, Sainio M, Jääskeläinen J. Population-based analysis of sporadic and type 2 neurofibromatosis-associated meningiomas and schwannomas. *Neurology*. 2000;54(1):71-76.

12. Evans DGR, Wallace A, Trueman L, Strachan T. Mosaicism in classical neurofibromatosis type 2: a common mechanism for sporadic disease in tumour prone syndromes? *Am J Hum Genet*. 1998;63:727-736.

13. Evans DGR, Ramsden RT, Shenton A, et al. Mosaicism in NF2 an update of risk based on uni/bilaterality of vestibular schwannoma at presentation and sensitive mutation analysis including MLPA. *J Med Genet*. 2007;44(7):424-428.

14. Kluwe L, Mautner VF, Heinrich B, et al. Molecular study of frequency of mosaicism in neurofibromatosis 2 patients with bilateral vestibular schwannomas. *J Med Genet*. 2003;40: 109-114.

15. Moyhuddin A, Baser ME, Watson C, et al. Somatic mosaicism in neurofibromatosis 2: prevalence and risk of disease transmission to offspring. *J Med Genet*. 2003;40:459-463.

16. Kanter WR, Eldridge R, Fabricant R, Allen JC, Koerber T. Central neurofibromatosis with bilateral acoustic neuroma. Genetic, clinical and biochemical distinctions from peripheral neurofibromatosis. *Neurology*. 1980;30:851-859.

17. Parry DM, Eldridge R, Kaiser-Kupfer MI, Bouzas EA, Pikus A, Patronas N. Neurofibromatosis 2 (NF2): clinical characteristics of 63 affected individuals and clinical evidence for heterogeneity. *Am J Med Genet*. 1994;52:450-451.

18. Mautner VF, Lindenau M, Baser ME, et al. The neuroimaging and clinical spectrum of neurofibromatosis 2. *Neurosurgery*. 1996;38: 880-885.

19. Evans DGR, Ramsden R, Birch J. Paediatric presentation of type 2 neurofibromatosis. *Arch Dis Child*. 1999;81:496-499.

20. Trivedi R, Byrne J, Huson SM, Donaghy M. Focal amyotrophy in neurofibromatosis 2. *J Neurol Neurosurg Psychiatry*. 2000;69(2):257-261.

21. Sperfeld AD, Hein C, Schroder JM, Ludolph AC, Hanemann CO. Occurrence and characterization of peripheral nerve involvement in neurofibromatosis type 2. *Brain*. 2002;125:996-1004.

22. Evans DGR, Newton V, Neary W, et al. Use of MRI and audiological tests in pre-symptomatic diagnosis of type 2 neurofibromatosis (NF2). *J Med Genet*. 2000;37:944-947.

23. King A, Biggs N, Ramsden RT, Wallace A, Gillespie J, Evans DGR. Spinal tumours in neurofibromatosis type 2: Is emerging knowledge of genotype predictive of natural history? *J Neurosurg Spine*. 2005;2(5):574-579.

24. Evans DGR, Baser ME, O'Reilly B, et al. Management of the patient and family with Neurofibromatosis 2: a consensus conference statement. *Brit J Neurosurg*. 2005;19:5-12.

25. Evans DGR, Ramsden RT, Shenton A, et al. Should NF2 mutation screening be undertaken in patients with an apparently isolated vestibular schwannoma? *Clin Genet*. 2007;71(4):354-358.

26. Evans DGR, Ramsden RT, Shenton A, et al. What are the implications in individuals with unilateral vestibular schwannoma and other neurogenic tumours? *J Neurosurg*. 2008;108(1):92-96.

27. Seizinger BR, Rouleau GA, Ozelius LG, et al. Genetic linkage of von Recklinghausen neurofibromatosis to the nerve growth factor receptor gene. *Cell*. 1987;49:589-594.

28. Rouleau G, Seizinger BR, Ozelius LG, et al. Genetic linkage analysis of bilateral acoustic neurofibromatosis to a DNA marker on chromosome 22. *Nature*. 1987;329:246-248.

29. Parry DM, MacCollin M, Kaiser-Kupfer MI, et al. Germ-line mutations in the neurofibromatosis 2 gene: correlations with disease severity and retinal abnormalities. *Am J Hum Genet*. 1996;59:529-539.

30. Ruttledge MH, Andermann AA, Phelan CM, et al. Type of mutation in the neurofibromatosis type 2 gene (NF2) frequently determines severity of disease. *Am J Hum Genet*. 1996;59:331-342.

31. Kluwe L, Bayer S, Baser ME, Hazim W, Haase W, Funsterer C. Mautner VF Identification of NF2 germ-line mutations and comparison with neurofibromatosis 2 phenotypes [published erratum in Hum Genet 1997;99(2):292]. *Hum Genet*. 1996;98:534-538.

32. Kluwe L, MacCollin M, Tatagiba M, et al. Phenotypic variability associated with 14 splice-site mutations in the NF2 gene. *Am J Med Genet*. 1998;77:228-233.

33. Evans DGR, Trueman L, Wallace A, Mason S, Strachan T. Genotype/phenotype correlations in type 2 neurofibromatosis:

evidence for more severe disease with truncating mutations. *J Med Genet*. 1998;35:450-455.

34. Baser ME, Kuramoto L, Joe H, et al. Genotype-phenotype correlations for nervous system tumours in neurofibromatosis 2: a population-based study. *Am J Hum Genet*. 2004;75:231-239.

35. Baser ME, Kuramoto L, Woods RH, et al. The location of constitutional neurofibromatosis 2 (NF2) splice-site mutations is associated with the severity of NF2. *J Med Genet*. 2005;42(7): 540-546.

36. Selvanathan SK, Shenton A, Ferner R, et al. Further genotype-phenotype correlations in neurofibromatosis type 2. *Clin Genet*. 2010;77(2):163-170.

37. Tsilchorozidou T, Menko F, Lalloo F, et al. Constitutional rearrangements of chromosome 22 as a cause of neurofibromatosis type 2. *J Med Genet*. 2004;41(7):529-534.

38. Kluwe L, Nygren AO, Errami A, et al. Screening for large mutations of the NF2 gene. *Genes Chromosomes Cancer*. 2005; 42(4):384-391.

39. MacCollin M, Chiocca EA, Evans DG, et al. Diagnostic criteria for schwannomatosis. *Neurology*. 2005;64(11):1838-1845.

40. Murray A, Hughes TAT, Neal JW, Howard E, Evans DGR, Harper PS. A case of multiple cutaneous schwannomas; schwannomatosis or neurofibromatosis type 2? *J Neurol Neurosurg Psychiatry*. 2006;77(2):269-271.

41. Baser ME, Friedman JM, Evans DG. Increasing the specificity of diagnostic criteria for schwannomatosis. *Neurology*. 2006;66(5): 730-732.

42. Hadfield KD, Newman WG, Bowers NL, et al. Molecular characterisation of SMARCB1 and NF2 in familial and sporadic schwannomatosis. *J Med Genet*. 2008;45(6):332-339.

43. Baser ME, Friedman JM, Wallace AJ, Ramsden RT, Joe H, Evans DGR. Evaluation of diagnostic criteria for neurofibromatosis 2. *Neurology*. 2002;59(11):1759-1765.

44. Evans DGR, Ramsden R, Huson SM, et al. Type 2 neurofibromatosis: the need for supraregional care. *J Laryngol Otol*. 1993; 107:401-406.

45. Slattery WH, Brackmann DE, Hitselberger W. Hearing preservation in neurofibromatosis type 2. *Am J Otol*. 1998;19:638-643.

46. Baser ME, Friedman JM, Aeschilman D, et al. Predictors of the risk of mortality in neurofibromatosis 2. *Am J Hum Genet*. 2002; 71:715-723.

47. Sobel RA, Wang Y. Vestibular (acoustic) schwannomas: histological features in neurofibromatosis 2 and in unilateral cases. *J Neuropathol Exp Neurol*. 1993;52:106-113.
48. Rowe JG, Radatz M, Walton L, Kemeny AA. Stereotactic radiosurgery for type 2 neurofibromatosis acoustic neuromas: patient selection and tumour size. *Stereotact Funct Neurosurg*. 2002;79:107-116.
49. Rowe JG, Radatz MW, Walton L, Soanes T, Rodgers J, Kemeny AA. Clinical experience with gamma knife stereotactic radiosurgery in the management of vestibular schwannomas secondary to type 2 neurofibromatosis. *J Neurol Neurosurg Psychiatry*. 2003;74(9):1288-1293.
50. Baser ME, Evans DGR, Jackler RK, Sujansky E, Rubenstein A. Malignant peripheral nerve sheath tumours, radiotherapy, and neurofibromatosis 2. *Br J Cancer*. 2000;82:998.
51. Evans DGR, Birch JM, Ramsden RT, Sharif S, Baser ME. Malignant transformation and new primary tumours after therapeutic radiation for benign disease: substantial risks in certain tumour-prone syndromes. *J Med Genet*. 2006;43(4):289-294.
52. Evans DG, Kalamarides M, Hunter-Schaedle K, et al. Consensus recommendations to accelerate clinical trials for neurofibromatosis type 2. *Clin Cancer Res*. 2009;15:5032-5039.
53. Hanemann CO. Magic but treatable? Tumours due to loss of merlin. *Brain*. 2008;131(pt 3):606-615.
54. Plotkin SR, Stemmer-Rachamimov AO, Barker FG 2nd, et al. Hearing improvement after bevacizumab in patients with neurofibromatosis type 2. *N Engl J Med*. 2009;361(4):358-367.
55. Mautner VF, Nguyen R, Kutta H, et al. Bevacizumab induces regression of vestibular schwannomas in patients with neurofibromatosis type 2. *Neuro Oncol*. 2010;12(1):14-18.
56. Parry DM, Eldridge R, Kaiser-Kupfer MI, Bouzas EA, Pikus A, Patronas N. Neurofibromatosis 2 (NF2): clinical characteristics of 63 affected individuals and clinical evidence for heterogeneity. *Am J Med Genet*. 1994;52:450-451.

Chapter 3
The Neurofibromatoses: Differential Diagnosis and Rare Subtypes

Susan M. Huson

Introduction

Accurate diagnosis of the type of neurofibromatosis is important for patient management and genetic counseling. In the majority of people with neurofibromatosis type one (NF1) and type two (NF2), the diagnosis is straightforward. In a specialist neurofibromatosis clinic, approximately 2% of new NF1 referrals will have an alternate non-NF diagnosis and 5% will have a specific NF subtype. This chapter reviews the differential diagnosis of and conditions related to NF1 and NF2.

The critical features used to differentiate the different types of NF are:

- The presence/absence of café au lait (CAL) spots with/without skin fold freckling
- The presence/distribution/histology of benign nerve tumors
- Eye features (often asymptomatic)

These disease features develop at different ages[1,2] (Table 3.1) – in NF1 the main feature in early childhood are the CAL spots which are nearly always obvious by age two. Conversely, in an adult the dermal neurofibromas become the key feature and CAL spots are known to become less obvious/decrease in number with age. With modern neuroimaging NF1 and

R.E. Ferner et al., *Neurofibromatoses in Clinical Practice*,
DOI: 10.1007/978-0-85729-629-0_3,
© Springer-Verlag London Limited 2011

TABLE 3.1. Distinguishing the major forms of neurofibromatosis: key features and age they develop.

NF Type	Gene/chromosome	Pigmentary changes	Peripheral nerve tumors	Ophthalmic features
NF1	*NF1/17*	*CAL spots*: most patients have ≥ 6 or more spots by their second birthday. Numbers increase to early teens but CAL fade and disappear in some adults *Skin-fold freckling*: tends to develop from around third birthday, usually obvious by early teens except the submammary freckles in women which develop as breasts enlarge	*Dermal (cutaneous) neurofibromas*: develop mainly from teens onward and are main cutaneous feature in adults. Present in majority of NF1 adults, who can have several hundred *Nodular (subcutaneous) neurofibromas*: subcutaneous lesions on peripheral nerves. Develop mainly from teens; present in only a proportion of patients (5–10%) *Plexiform neurofibromas*: externally visible plexiform neurofibromas present in 25–30% patients, usually obvious by age 10 and major disfiguring lesions on face by 3 years, elsewhere by 5 years	*Lisch nodules*: develop during childhood and present in ~95% adult patients

Legius syndrome	SPRED1/15	Exactly the same as in NF1	NONE	NONE
NF2	NF2(MERLIN)/22	*CAL spots*: present in 43% of cases in one large series BUT only 1% had six; 24% had one spot, 11% had two spots, and 7% had 3 or 4	*Overall*: Peripheral Schwannomas present in 68% of patients BUT only 10% have >10 and in one large study maximum number was 27	Lens opacities/cataracts
		Skin-fold freckling: not seen in NF2	*NF2 plaques*: present in 48% of patients and develop from early childhood	Amblyopia (no obvious cause)
			Peripheral nerve schwannomas: present in 43%	Astrocytic hamartomas
			Dermal (cutaneous) schwannomas: look exactly like dermal neurofibromas in NF1, present in 27% but in much lower numbers than in NF1	Combined retinal and retinal pigment epithelium hamartomas
Schwannomatosis	INI1/SMARCB1/22	NONE	*Peripheral nerve and spinal nerve root schwannomas*: usually develop from teens onward	NONE

NF2 are rarely confused in adults but NF1 is often the first diagnosis considered in children presenting with NF2-related skin changes. Very occasionally a major NF1 complication may present before the CAL spots are obvious – I have met parents who have been accused of nonaccidental injury prior to the correct diagnosis of tibial pseudarthrosis been made.

Although molecular genetic testing is now available for NF1 and NF2, for neither condition is mutation detection 100% and the presence of genetic mosaicism in sporadic cases complicates the situation further.[3-6] Prior to any molecular testing full clinical evaluation, with radiological and histological review if indicated is essential. In patients where things do not fit together, review in a specialist NF clinic may be of benefit prior to any molecular genetic testing.

Case History: The Importance of Clinical Diagnosis Prior to Genetic Testing

A 14-year-old girl was referred for genetic assessment with possible NF1. The previous year she had several tongue lesions removed which were reported as neurofibromas and the question of NF1 raised. Around the same time she had had some eye problems and thickened corneal nerves noted coincidentally. She was referred for pediatric assessment. She had one CAL spot. NF1 gene testing was requested and no mutation identified. She was then referred for genetic assessment.

There was no significant family history. The preoperative pictures of her tongue lesions showed multiple small papillomatous lesions. On examination the only skin feature was the CAL spot but she was thin with hyperextensible joints and prominent lips. She had an asymmetrically enlarged thyroid gland. A clinical diagnosis of MEN 2B was made and this was confirmed by the finding of the M918T mutation in the *RET* proto-oncogene. Investigations and subsequent surgery diagnosed metastatic medullary thyroid carcinoma.

Key Points

- The tongue is not a common site for small neurofibromas in NF1; plexiform lesions of the area show diffuse enlargement of the tongue.
- One CAL spot is within normal limits.
- Thickened corneal nerves are classically associated with multiple endocrine neoplasia type 2B not NF1.

Clinical Assessment

The points I highlight in this section are those that assist in establishing the type of NF. Some patients will have clinical symptoms/signs that take clinical priority – for example a patient with NF1, NF2, or schwannomatosis may present with symptoms/signs of cord compression which requires urgent assessment. Even then it is usually possible to diagnose the type of NF during the same assessment and this allows perioperative planning, for example, in sporadic cases of NF2 and schwannomatosis collection of fresh frozen tissue for DNA analysis is helpful. Figure 3.1 shows a flow chart to aid in assessing a child with multiple CAL spots.

Past Medical History

Regardless of the age of the patient, I find it useful to take a full medical and social history from birth onward. This builds up a picture of the age of appearance of key disease features, any major medical problems, and whether learning and behavior problems have been an issue.

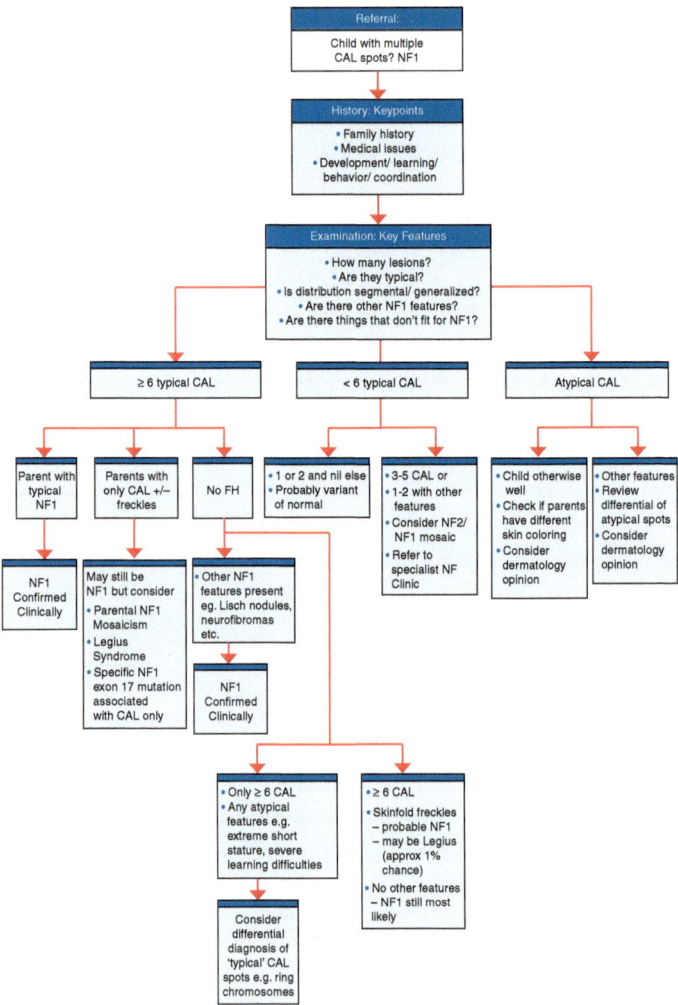

FIGURE 3.1. Diagnostic approach to a child with multiple CAL spots.

Family History

In both NF1 and NF2 approximately 50% of patients are the first in their families and the diseases are fully penetrant (so they do not "skip" generations in the pedigree[6]). Recording the family tree, going back to the grandparents of the index case, allows you to:

- Build up a picture of the family's experience of the disease.
- Identify which family members need assessing.
- Identify any unusual features – for example, affected siblings/cousins with NF1 and unaffected parents are very unusual. Prior to the recognition of the constitutional mismatch repair deficiency phenotype (CMMR-D, which is discussed later in the chapter[7]), several of the families had been presumed to have NF1 because of multiple CAL spots in one or more sibs/cousins. In retrospect the clues to the alternate diagnosis were the family history of cancers seen in hereditary nonpolyposis colon cancer and consanguinity.

Examination

The main systems that assist in the differential diagnosis are examination of the skin, eyes, and nervous system; in possible NF1 this is complemented by checking for disease complications that may be present in a patient of that age. In assessing NF-related skin pigmentation, an ultraviolet light is rarely necessary other than in very pale skinned people. Eye examination needs to be done by an Ophthalmologist familiar with NF – a slit lamp is needed to distinguish Lisch nodules from the iris nevus and the lens opacities in NF2 are often only seen by slit lamp.[8]

Radiology/Histology Review

In atypical cases the value of having radiology and histology reviewed by colleagues familiar with NF cannot be understated. Radiologists familiar with neurofibromatosis may pick up subtle features on review which point to the subtype. Neurofibromas and schwannomas can often not be differentiated clinically or radiologically and then histology is vital.

NF Pigmentary Changes: Key Clinical Features

Café au Lait Spots

CAL spots or patchy pigmentation of other kinds[9] are listed as features of a large number of genetic syndromes, of which NF1 is by far the most common. What is important clinically is to ensure that what are being labeled as CAL spots are typical for NF1. Figure 3.2 shows different kinds of CAL pigmentation. The key features of CAL in NF1 are[6,9]:

- Macular (flat), any lesion with any thickening is not a CAL spot.
- They usually have an oval shape with a smooth edge and the pigmentation is uniform within the spot.
- In pale skinned individuals they are coffee colored, whereas in dark skinned individuals they may be dark brown or black.
- They may be present at birth but more usually develop in the first few months of life and are nearly always obvious by the second birthday.
- They grow with the child, becoming larger with age.
- They can occur anywhere on the body but are mainly seen on the trunk and limbs; they are rarely found on the face, scalp, palms, and soles.
- Very small, nonsignificant patches are not counted; the NF1 diagnostic criteria use specific sizes for inclusion, which is measured across the maximum diameter of the lesion: in prepubertal lesion spots of >5 mm are counted and in post-pubertal >1.5 cm.
- The spots tend to be 2–5 cm in diameter but can be larger. If a patient has a much larger area it needs to be monitored as this can be a marker for an area where a plexiform will develop.

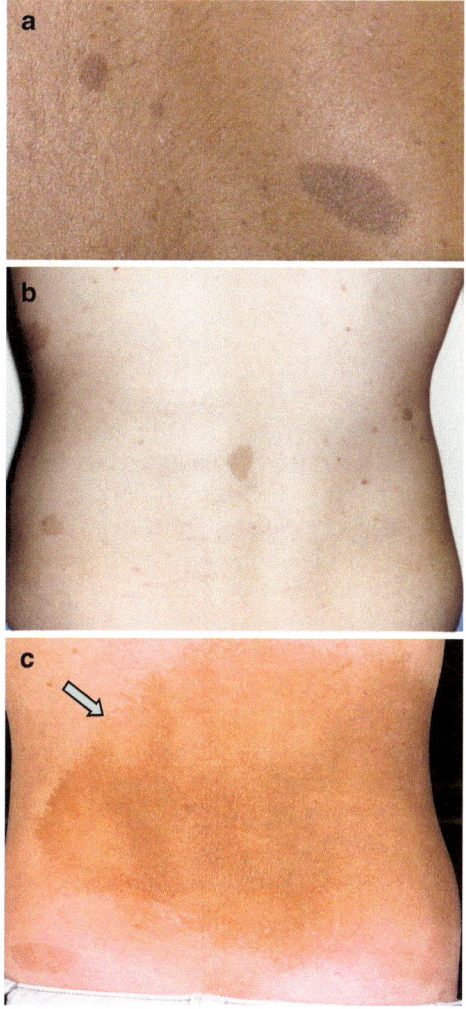

FIGURE 3.2. Different kinds of CAL pigmentation (**a**) Typical NF1 CAL spots in an Asian patient: note relatively smooth outline and even pigmentation. (**b**) CAL spots in a patient with Legius syndrome, exactly the same as in NF1 (reproduced with permission from Spurlock et al.[10]). (**c**) Large CAL with irregular outline and hypertrichosis overlying a large internal plexiform neurofibroma. (**d**) Atypical CAL lesion in an Asian child with ataxia telangiectasia: note irregular outline and uneven depth of pigmentation.

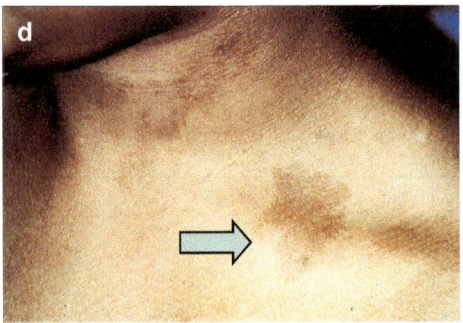

FIGURE 3.2. (continued).

- The NF1 diagnostic criteria require 6 or more CAL spots and NF1 children often have many more; 10% of the general population have one or two CAL spots. When children present with 3–5 CAL spots (which is uncommon) I usually monitor them through childhood because of the rare possibility they have NF2 or are one of the rare cases of NF1 with <6 CAL.
- NF1 CAL spots have no distinguishing pathological features; biopsy is not a helpful aid to diagnosis.
- CAL spots become paler and can disappear with age.
- CAL spots are not at risk of malignant change and their number does not correlate with disease severity in any way.
- Although patients with NF2 have CAL spots more frequently than the general population, it is very unusual for them to have six or more (1%) and they do not get skin fold freckling.

Skin Fold Freckling

Why NF1 patients develop freckles in very specific areas of the body remains unexplained but clinically it is an important aid to diagnosis. The freckles, like the CAL spots, never do any harm but are an important diagnostic feature. They develop after the CAL, usually from around the 3rd birthday and can affect the axillae, base of the neck, and groins. Women may develop them below the breasts and overweight people in skin folds. Some patients develop freckles over their whole trunk.

Peripheral Nerve Tumors in NF: Clinical Clues to Diagnosis

Neurofibromas Versus Schwannomas

The important thing to remember in assessing lesions in patients referred as "query form of NF," is that it is not possible to distinguish individual neurofibromas and schwannomas clinically (Fig. 3.3). As reviewed in Chap. 1, the appearance and problems associated with neurofibromas are dependent on where in the nervous system they develop (dermal (cutaneous),

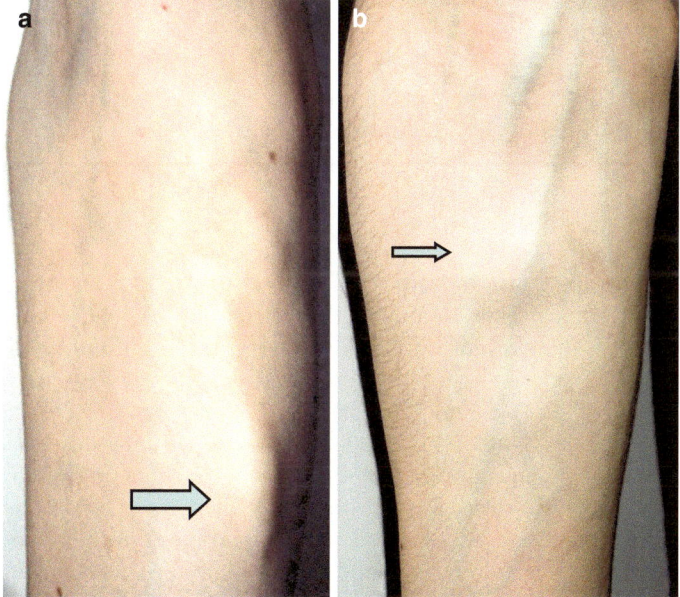

FIGURE 3.3. Peripheral nerve lesions (arrowed) in the forearm: (**a**) The patient has NF1 (neurofibromas); (**b**) the patient has NF2 (schwannomas) – clinically they are indistinguishable.

peripheral nerve, or spinal nerve root). Schwannomas in NF2 at the different sites present very much like neurofibromas. The only tumor that virtually always has a unique appearance is the NF2 plaque lesion described in the next section.

The problem in distinguishing neurofibromas and schwannomas clinically is usually not an issue as other diagnostic features of the type of NF will be present. The times when it becomes important are in assessing patients with segmental/mosaic phenotypes presenting with just localized nerve involvement when histology is usually necessary. The other cases that can cause confusion are cases with NF2 and marked skin involvement. These tend to be people with severe NF2 with no family history where dermal or peripheral nerve lesions present before cranial or spinal lesions. Although schwannomas are not seen in NF1, neurofibromas can occasionally occur in NF2 or tumors with a mixed neurofibroma/schwannoma picture are reported. Rare patients with severe NF2 can develop plexiform lesions in childhood and these too are indistinguishable from those in NF1 clinically, although are usually plexiform schwannomas histologically. The clues clinically are the reduced number or lack of CAL spots, specific eye signs, and identification of NF2 plaques if present.

NF2 Plaques

These are the one specific cutaneous lesion that are an invaluable clinical clue.[11] Initially they can look like small CAL spots – the skin has a brown–orange color; the difference is that the skin is slightly thickened and there is often excessive hair growth (see Fig. 2.10, Chap. 2). They rarely grow beyond 1–2 cm in diameter. Histologically they are usually described as having "schwannomatous elements." When a child presents with an NF2-related eye problem, isolated peripheral nerve amyotrophy or NF2-related cranial or spinal tumor, clinical examination for NF2 plaques is essential. The youngest patient I have seen with one was 18 months; they presented with unilateral amblyopia and a dysplastic optic disk which was recognized by an Ophthalmologist familiar with NF2.

Eye Features of NF

The eye features in the main forms of NF are summarized in Table 3.1. As mentioned above, the critical thing here is to ensure that patients are being assessed by an Ophthalmologist familiar with the different forms of NF.[8] Although a few NF1 patients have so many Lisch nodules that can be seen by ophthalmoscope, one cannot rely on just ophthalmoscopic examination to say they are absent.

NF1 Differential Diagnosis: The NF1/NF2 Overlap

The reasons NF1 and NF2 were lumped together historically are because of overlapping skin features and the difficulty in distinguishing, both clinically and radiologically, neurofibromas and schwannomas. It is very unusual for people with NF1 to be diagnosed as having NF2, but "?NF1" is often the initial diagnosis in children presenting with NF2-related skin changes. The key things to check here are:

- Are there any NF2 plaques?
- An ophthalmic examination
- Histology review of any lesions removed if described as neurofibromas

Why early recognition of NF2 is important is because the NF2-related VS can get to a considerable size before causing hearing loss. I have seen numerous patients diagnosed in their late teens, presenting with significant brain stem compression, who have either had ophthalmic review for NF2-related problems in early childhood or who have had skin lesions removed over the years, the significance of which were not appreciated.

When I began working with NF families in the 1980s, misdiagnosis between NF1 and NF2 was common. Fortunately with increased awareness and improved neuroimaging the situation has improved. Despite this, within the last 5 years, patients under our care have been misinformed by colleagues. For example, a man with NF2 and multiple dermal (cutaneous) schwannomas was told he must have NF1 and NF2 and the possibility of NF2 was queried in a girl with severe spinal nerve root involvement and NF1. The patient was so alarmed by this that we had to undertake genetic testing to provide reassurance.

Case History: Delay in Diagnosis in a Child with NF2

A 10-year-old boy was referred with a diagnosis of possible NF2. There was no family history. He had been reviewed for various cutaneous lesions since the age of 5 in dermatology, pediatrics, and plastic surgery. He only had 2 CAL spots and NF1 had been thought to be unlikely. The lesions removed were initially reported as neurofibromas; however, at the age of 9 a lesion was removed and was thought to be atypical for a neurofibroma. Expert review diagnosed a plexiform schwannoma. The possibility of NF2 was considered.

Cutaneous examination showed several NF2 plaques and nodular (subcutaneous) peripheral nerve lesions. His first cranial scan showed bilateral vestibular schwannomas of significant size; despite this, he had only just started to notice any hearing problems. Mutation testing identified a nonsense mutation in the NF2 gene.

Key Points

- Dermal (cutaneous) and peripheral nerve lesions in the absence of ≥6 CAL spots make NF2 a real possibility.
- The vestibular schwannomas in NF2 can grow to a considerable size and not affect hearing.
- The NF2 plaque is an invaluable diagnostic feature in childhood.
- If the tumor histology does not fit the clinical picture, ask for review.

NF1 Subtypes

Introduction

These are all caused by germline or somatic mutations in the *NF1* gene except Legius syndrome, which is caused by mutations in another RasMAPK gene, *SPRED1*. The importance of recognizing the different types is that they have either specific genetic implications (e.g., the much lower recurrence risk in segmental NF1) or a different natural history (e.g., very mild in the CAL-only phenotypes, consistently more severe in microdeletion patients and spinal NF1). At most these subtypes probably account for around 10% of the NF1 group. In the majority of families NF1 is extremely variable in its manifestations even WITHIN the family.

Segmental/Localized NF1

The term segmental or localized NF1 is used to describe the patients with disease features limited to one or more body segments. The estimated disease prevalence is between 1 in 36,000–40,000 individuals in the general population.[12] Most patients are asymptomatic and seek medical opinion because of the unusual appearance of the skin. In the majority of patients the area involved is unilateral and varies in size from a narrow strip to one quadrant and occasionally one half of the body. Some patients have more than one segment involved on both sides of the midline, either in a symmetrical or asymmetrical arrangement. Within the affected area the patients either have NF1-related pigmentary changes, neurofibromas alone, or both. Patients may also present with isolated plexiform neurofibromas and no other disease features.

NF1-related pigmentary changes are the most common phenotype. In a number of patients the whole segment of affected skin is darker and within this CAL spots and freckles develop. The segment of pigmented skin may be the presenting feature in infants and the NF1 changes develop within the segment with time.

The frequency of NF1 complications is much lower in segmental cases (only 7% in one series[12]). If the phenotype includes neurofibromas on major peripheral nerves or a major plexiform there is still a risk of malignant change.

In the Manchester clinic we offer annual review until late teens and then adjust follow-up according to phenotype. If there is internal involvement of significance we follow as we would in generalized NF1. We advise uncomplicated patients that the risk of associated problems is low, but if unusual symptoms develop always to ensure the Doctor they are seeing is aware of their segmental NF1 diagnosis.

Genetically, the phenotype results from somatic mutation in the NF1 gene, with the manifestations depending on the timing of mutation in embryonic development. The importance of recognizing this group is for their different natural history and because they have much lower recurrence risks in offspring. In my own practice I use an empiric recurrence risk of 5% at most, unless the portion of the body affected is particularly large. It is exceptional to find a mosaic gene mutation on analysis of lymphocytes and it is usually necessary to perform NF1 mutation analysis in schwann cells derived from neurofibromas or melanocytes from the CAL spots of the affected segment to identify the causal mutation.[13] From a clinical viewpoint, patients with segmental NF1 sometimes find the small, but definite risk of a child with generalized NF1 too big a risk. In these cases mutation analysis on affected tissue can define the mutation so that prenatal testing can be offered.

When counseling parents of a child with newly diagnosed NF1 about recurrence risks, it is my practice to examine the skin and irides of the parents. Most affected parents report their skin changes, even though they may not have been formally diagnosed before. However, I have very occasionally found areas of segmental NF1 change the significance of which the parent had not appreciated. If the parent's examination is completely normal, then I give a recurrence risk of much less than 1%. There have been very few reported cases of pure gonadal mosaicism in NF1[4]; in my own practice I have seen only one family with two affected children and we found they had different NF1 mutations.

Generalized Mosaic NF1

As Professor Evans reviews in his chapter on NF2, up to one third of sporadic cases of NF2 are mosaics, presenting with mild disease which is more usually generalized than limited to a body area. One of the ways the significance of mosaicism in NF2 was highlighted was that the number of affected children born to sporadic cases was less than the expected 50%.[14] Although early NF1 studies such as my own[15] found no evidence of this in NF1, the general awareness of NF1 at the time was so limited that one would only expect sporadic cases with very obvious NF1 to be diagnosed. The other pointer to a higher frequency of mosaic cases is a lower mutation detection rate in sporadic cases than in the second generation of familial cases; although NF1 series have given conflicting results to date (reviewed in Kehrer-Sawatski and Cooper[4] and Ruggieri and Huson[12]) this could still be due to only obviously affected sporadic cases being tested. Mosaicism in sporadic NF1 microdeletion cases, particularly type two deletions, is well recognized.[16] With improved mutation detection techniques and awareness of the importance of recognizing mosaicism for genetic counseling, it is likely more cases of nondeletion sporadic NF1 will be found to be mosaics. Muram-Zborovski et al.[17] report a father and son with only CAL spots who they thought may have Legius syndrome. Molecular analysis showed no SPRED1 mutations, that the boy had an NF1 mutation which his father was mosaic for on lymphocyte analysis.

The NF1 Microdeletion Syndrome

Up to 5% of NF1 mutations are large deletions of both the *NF1* and a variable number of flanking genes. The clinical importance of the deletions is that they are associated with a more consistently severe phenotype. Clear delineation of genotype/phenotype has been hampered as some reports contain detailed molecular analysis with limited clinical detail and vice versa. Fortunately with larger studies[18,19] and studies which include a review of all previously

TABLE 3.2. Clinical features associated with the common
type one NF1 microdeletion.

Feature	Frequency/comment
Dysmorphic facial features: hypertelorism, downslanting palpebral fissures, broad fleshy nose, "coarse" face becoming more marked with age	26/29[19]
Overgrowth with tall stature and large hands and feet	13/28[19]
Other dysmorphic features	
Pectus excavatum	9/29[19]
Broad neck	9/29
Excess soft tissue in hands and feet	12/24
Musculoskeletal features	
Joint hyperflexibility	21/29[19]
Muscular hypotonia	13/29
Bone cysts	8/16
Pes cavus	5/29 (only reported in Mautner series[19])
Neurofibroma burden	Dermal (cutaneous) neurofibromas consistently reported to occur at an earlier age and in increased numbers Mautner et al. report increased frequency of all types of neurofibroma compared with general NF1 population including spinal neurofibromas
MPNST	6/29[19]; De Raedt et al.[23] estimate double lifetime risk of general NF1 population
Learning and development	Significant delay in cognitive development 14/29 with IQ < 70 in 8/21[19] Learning difficulties 13/29 Mean IQ lower than general NF1 population by 12.5 points (76 in microdeletions compared with 88.5[24])
Other features which may occur in excess	Congenital heart disease[21,22] Scoliosis[19]

Source: Data compiled from Mautner et al.,[19] Venturin et al.,[21] Mensink et al.,[22] De Raedt et al.[23] and Descheemaeker et al.[24]

published cases[20-22], the phenotype, particularly for the common, type one, deletion is evolving (Table 3.2, Fig. 3.4). There have also been additional studies comparing one particular aspect of the deletion phenotype with the general NF1 population – IQ, growth, and frequency of MPNST.[23-25]

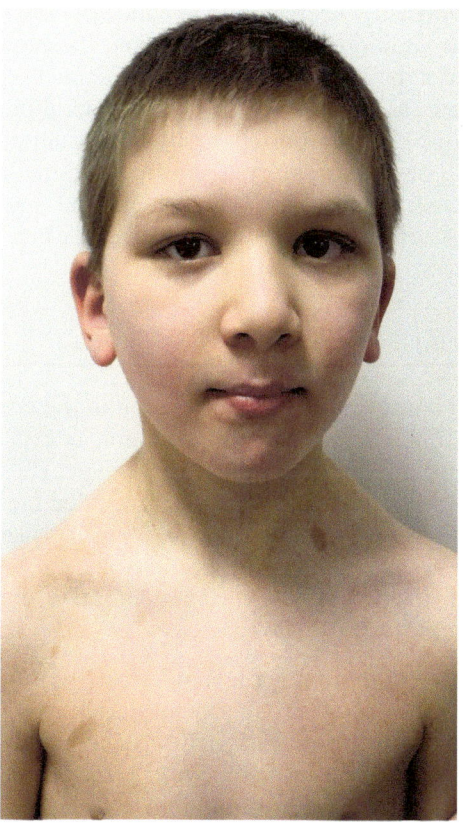

FIGURE 3.4. A child with a NF1 microdeletion: note the broad nasal bridge, slight downslanting palpebral fissures, low set ears, and high trapezius insertion giving appearance of broad neck.

Molecular Basis of Deletions

At a molecular level there are three recurrent deletions.[18] The most common type one deletion is a 1.4 Mb deletion with 14 additional genes deleted, caused by nonallelic homologous recombination between two regions of low copy repeats; these deletions are rarely mosaic. Type two deletions are often mosaic, and there is a 1.2 Mb deletion with 13 additional genes. The deletion is caused by recombination between the *SUZ12* gene and its pseudogene which are on opposite sides of the NF1 gene. The smallest recurrent deletions (type three) have only recently been identified[18] and are only 1 Mb in size with eight additional deleted genes and the breakpoints lie within the same distal but a different proximal region of low copy repeats as the type one deletions. In addition there are a number of patients reported with atypical, unique deletions of varying sizes. Laboratory-based studies estimate microdeletion account for 5–10% of NF1 patients but this may represent overascertainment of severely affected cases.

The Clinical Phenotype

The most consistent phenotype is seen in the common type one deletion.[18-22] Mosaicism is common in type two deletions and can result in a milder phenotype. The phenotype of the three initial type three cases included facial dysmorphism. The value of these and other atypical cases will be in assessing which flanking gene contributes to a particular disease feature. The most consistent features associated with deletions are:

- *Facial dysmorphism*: Three large series[19,21,22] have reported a much increased frequency of facial dysmorphism in microdeletion cases than in the general NF1 population (52–78% compared with 5–15%). However, all these series included either cases from multiple clinicians or a literature review and mainly combine data from all kinds of deletion. In a large series of type one cases from a single clinic, Mautner et al.[19] report facial dysmorphism in 26/29 cases

(90%). The main features are downslanting palpebral fissures, hypertelorism, ptosis, and a broad fleshy nose (Fig. 3.4). The overall dysmorphic facial appearance is described as coarse and this becomes more marked with age.

- *Developmental delay and learning problems*: Microdeletion patients are often ascertained because their degree of developmental delay and subsequent intellectual development is more severe than in NF1 as a whole. The NF1 deletion children often exhibit delayed early motor milestones, which is unusual in nondeleted patients. One study[24] looked specifically at type one deletion patients and found a full scale IQ difference of 12.5 points compared with a nonmicrodeletion group (mean IQ 76 in microdeletion group and 88.5 in nondeletion group). In their series of type one patients, Mautner et al.[19] reported significant delay in cognitive development in 14/29, with a further 13 patients having learning problems. Of the 21 who had formal IQ measurements, the mean IQ was almost the same as in the Belgium study (76.9), with 8/21 (38%) having an IQ <70. They also report a possible increase in muscular hypotonia (45%) and speech difficulties (48%).
- In series where CNS imaging is available there has been a suggestion of an increased frequency of structural brain anomalies.[19,26]
- *Excessive neurofibroma burden and MPNST*: From the earliest reports of deletions one of the major features was that patients tended to have early onset of appearance and excessive numbers of neurofibromas.[22] This has always been my clinical impression but data from two recent large series are conflicting. Mautner et al.[19] report an increased frequency of all types of neurofibromas: cutaneous, subcutaneous, plexiform, and spinal. Whereas Pasmant et al.[18] reporting on a large multicentre cohort found no significant increase compared with nondeleted patients. My own clinical experience would support Mautner's findings, in that 3 of 15 cases ascertained through the Oxford NF clinic had had surgery for cervical nerve root neurofibromas and our adult microdeletion patients have all had a large dermal neurofibroma burden.

- Patients with the common microdeletions are also at an elevated risk of MPNST. The lifetime risk of MPNST in NF1 as a whole is in the region of 8–13%; De Raedt et al.[23] estimated that the deletion patients have double this risk. In the Mautner series,[19] 6/29 (21%) type one deletion cases had developed MPNST.

- *Cardiovascular abnormalities*: A variety of congenital heart problems have been reported in cases with typical deletion sizes, including atrial and ventricular septal defects, patent ductus arteriosus, pulmonary stenosis, dilated aortic valve, hypertrophic cardiomyopathy, and mitral valve prolapse.[21] However, no one specific lesion has emerged as being more frequent in the larger series and so it is difficult to know their significance.[18,19] However, there is enough concern to warrant careful cardiac examination, even in the absence of symptoms. One of the patients reported by Mensink et al. developed bacterial endocarditis in previously undiagnosed mitral valve prolapse.[22]

- *Stature*: Another feature that makes many deletion cases stand out in the NF1 clinic is the fact they are taller than average. In my Welsh population study, 31.5% of patients were at or below the third centile for height and we showed that the NF1 children were 7–8 cm shorter than their affected siblings. In contrast 19/114 reported deletion cases[22] had tall stature/overgrowth. In the Mautner series,[19] 46% of the patients were ≥94th centile for height. Spiegel et al.[25] showed the growth of their cohort (19 with a type one and two with a type two deletion) of deleted patients showed a distinct pattern of childhood overgrowth. They speculated that a gene associated with overgrowth lay within the deletion. This was subsequently proven by the finding of mutations in *RNF135* in individuals with significant overgrowth who did not have NF1.[27] In the Pasmant series the four patients whose deletion excluded RNF135 were not overgrown.[18]

- *Other skeletal and connective tissue features*: The patients with deletions who were tall in the Mautner series also had large hands and feet.[19] In the same series 5/29 patients had pes cavus which had not previously been reported. The other probable new association was of an increased frequency of bone cysts. In their case series and literature review, Mensink reported large hands and feet in 25/114 cases.[22] The palms of the hands were soft and fleshy with an excess of connective tissue in half of Mautner's series. Joint hypermobility also seems to be commoner in the deletion cases (72 and 58% frequency in two large series[19,22]). Other skeletal features that probably occur more frequently in the deletion patients are pectus excavatum and a broad neck with downslanting shoulders.[19,22]

- Scoliosis may also be more common in deletion cases than in the general NF1 population although the data, even from large series, are conflicting.

Should All NF1 Patients Be Tested for Deletions?

In the Manchester clinic at the present time we do not offer routine mutation testing. If a patient has any dysmorphic or other clinical features which suggest a deletion we recommend testing. However, the series of Mautner et al.[19] highlights that even within the same type one deletions there is variability and a case could be made that all newly diagnosed patients should be checked for a deletion. I endorse the conclusions of Mautner et al.[19] that once identified this group of NF1 patients require increased clinical and psychological support.

Spinal NF1

The importance of recognition of this rare NF1 subtype[28-36] is because of the consistent presence of multiple spinal neurofibromas, usually bilateral and involving all 38 spinal nerve roots, which is extremely uncommon in ordinary NF1 (Fig. 3.5). In most NF1 families, just one person will develop a symptomatic spinal tumor, whereas in spinal NF1, the phenotype has largely been consistent in reported families. Furthermore, in spinal NF1 there may be marked involvement of major peripheral nerves – MPNST have been reported both in spinal and peripheral nerve lesions in these patients.[28,33]

FIGURE 3.5. A maximum intensity projection reformat of a coronal STIR whole body acquisition whole body MRI of a patient with spinal neurofibromatosis: note extensive involvement of spinal nerve roots and major peripheral nerves.

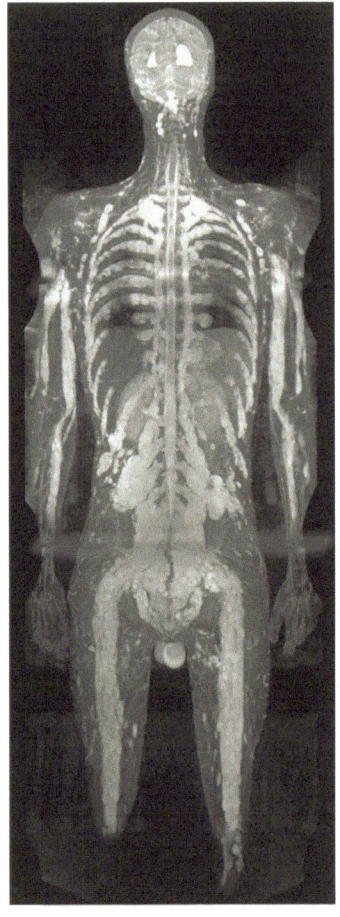

The other consistent feature in the reported families has been that other major NF1 features and complications are usually absent. The exception to this is café au lait spots, although some cases have ≤6 and no skinfold freckling. Dermal (cutaneous) neurofibromas are usually absent. However, peripheral nerve involvement can be marked with patients having multiple nodular (subcutaneous) neurofibromas along their course – this can be particularly obvious along the intercostal nerves.

In our own clinic we do whole-body MRI in patients with a suggestive phenotype, proceeding to spinal MRI in those with the phenotype. These patients require close neurological monitoring and have open access to our clinic for any new/changing symptoms. The role of follow-up scans is being determined; at present we are doing two yearly scans or earlier if new signs/symptoms develop.

The molecular basis for this phenotype is still to be elucidated; its existence suggests that the requirement for development of dermal (cutaneous) and spinal lesions may be different. However, consistently, in the reported cases there has been an excess of splice site and missense mutations.[32,35,36] One hypothesis proposed was that these mutations may result in abnormal protein production with a "dominant-negative effect."[30] This cannot be the sole explanation as a number of similar mutations have been reported in patients with typical NF1.[36] Other suggestions have been that of a closely linked modifier gene.[34] The recent report of excess numbers of spinal neurofibromas in microdeletion patients adds some support to this.[19,36] There has also been one family which did not map to the NF1 locus suggesting genetic heterogeneity.[28]

Watson Syndrome

Watson[37] described autosomal dominant inheritance of pulmonary stenosis, multiple café au lait spots, and intelligence at the lower end of the normal range. At that time pulmonary stenosis was not recognized as an NF1 complication and all family members had mild learning problems which is unusual in NF1. A few similar families have since been reported. Follow-up of the original Watson patients confirmed that their phenotype had remained distinct from NF1.[38] Although a few individuals had Lisch nodules on slit lamp examination and some had developed neurofibromas, both of these features were present at a very much lower frequency than is usually seen in NF1. Since then three different mutations in the NF1 gene have been reported in Watson syndrome (an 80-kb deletion, an inframe tandem duplication in exon

28, and the exon 17 3-bp deletion discussed below[39,40], respectively). This suggests that the NF1 mutation alone is not sufficient to explain this distinctive phenotype.

CAL-Only Phenotypes

Riccardi[41] first described families with CAL spots in numbers comparable to NF1, but without Lisch nodules and neurofibromas, although pectus excavatum and nonspecific learning problems did occur. Clinically therefore one can only make the diagnosis in the presence of two or more affected generations. Even then there is the possibility that a mildly affected sporadic parent could be a mosaic. This was therefore a phenotype for which molecular genetic testing has long been awaited.

Two specific and separate genetic mechanisms have now been identified. One is a specific mutation in exon 17 of the *NF1* gene[42] (exon 17 using NF consortium nomenclature; exon 22 using National Center for Biotechnology Information nomenclature) and the other mutations in another gene in the same cellular pathway, SPRED1 on chromosome 15[43] have now been identified associated with this phenotype. The CAL-only phenotypes are relatively uncommon, even in a large NF1 clinic. The importance of recognition for families is the much better natural history, with the removal of most of the concerns associated with NF1 (e.g., How many dermal neurofibromas will develop? What complications can happen?).

Legius Syndrome

Legius syndrome is the most important cause of the "familial CAL" phenotype identified to date. No affected individuals have been reported with any form of neurofibroma or Lisch nodules. Affected individuals have a higher frequency of learning problems than the general population but these have been milder and less frequent than seen in NF1. No consistent association with specific malignancies has emerged so far; the reported tumors are listed in Table 3.3.

TABLE 3.3. Summary of clinical features of reported cases of Legius syndrome.

Feature	Frequency/comment/references if not compiled from all
Age (years)	
≥18	54/106
≥20	14/40 (Messiaen et al.[44] use a 20 year cut-off)
Familial/sporadic/unknown	129/13/4
CAL spots	
Present	142/146
Adults with ≥6 CAL >1.5 cm diameter	39/61[10, 43-46]
Children with ≥6 CAL >0.5 cm	60/64[43-47]
Skinfold freckling	62/146
Neurofibromas of any sort	0
Lisch nodules	0
Macrocephaly	9/100; two papers record true and relative macrocephaly in 10/55[44,46]; in one series head circumference on higher centile than height in 20/24[46]
Learning and behavior	
Learning difficulties	26/142 (data from Denayer et al.[46])
Delayed psychomotor development (mostly confined to speech delay)	13/142
Hyperactivity, attention problems, or ADHD	14/142
Dysmorphic features	
Noonan-like facies	13/146
Pectus excavatum	13/146
Postaxial polydactyly (unilateral)	3/146
Excess periorbital pigmentation	1/146 (only reported in one case[10])

(continued)

TABLE 3.3. (continued).

Feature	Frequency/comment/references if not compiled from all
Tumors	
Lipomas	19/146 plus 1 angiolipoma
Single case tumors of uncertain significance as yet	Childhood acute myeloblastic leukemia; abdominal wall desmoid; vestibular schwannoma (patient aged >50); tenosynovial giant cell tumor; ovarian dermoid tumor; nonsmall cell lung cancer; childhood renal cancer (possibly Wilms); colon adenoma (45 years)
Other reported features which can occur in NF1	Scoliosis – four cases reported in series of Denayer et al.[46] but no detailed description Congenital pulmonary stenosis and mitral valve prolapse (same patient[44]) T2 hyperintensities on cranial MRI – reported in a 39 and 11-year-old[46]
Other reported features which can be seen in other RASopathies (one case each)	Inguinal hemangioma[10]; temporal venous anomaly[44]; vascular anomaly leg[44]

Source: Data compiled from Brems et al.,[43] Spurlock et al.,[10] Pasmant et al.,[45] Messiaen et al.,[44] Muram-Zborovski et al.[47] and Denayer et al.[46]

The syndrome was first reported as an "NF1-like syndrome"[43] but has now been named Legius syndrome to reflect its clinical and molecular characterization by the group of Professor Eric Legius and the absence of neurofibromas. In the large Leuven NF1 clinic Professor Legius identified five families with CAL spots, axillary freckling, macrocephaly, and Noonan-like facies in some individuals. No neurofibromas or Lisch nodules were present. *NF1* mutations were not identified in these families and linkage studies in the two largest families mapped the locus to chromosome 15. In this region *SPRED1* was recognized as an ideal candidate, as it negatively regulates MAPK signaling like neurofibromin. Mutations were found in all five families. They then extended their studies to 86 unrelated patients who had negative NF1 testing and CAL spots +/− freckling only and found 7/86 (8%) had *SPRED1* mutations.

The consistency of the phenotype and the significance of Legius syndrome as a cause of multiple CAL has since been determined through reports from several centers[10,44-47] (Table 3.3). The CAL spots and freckles seen in Legius are exactly the same in appearance and age of onset as in NF1 (Fig. 3.2). A small proportion of individuals with the mutation have had <6 CAL spots; the majority of these cases were adults and four cases have had none (3 adults aged 60, 58, and 37 and a child aged 2 years[43,44,46]). Therefore on assessing families it is important to test both parents of sporadic cases and in any family to offer testing to at-risk individuals with any CAL spots.

Of the 146 reported cases none have had any form of neurofibroma and those examined have not had Lisch nodules. Learning problems, speech delay, and ADHD are associated but at a lower frequency than in NF1. It should be noted that one report of a SPRED1 mutation in a child with an orbital plexiform and sphenoid wing dysplasia has subsequently been retracted as the child did not have a mutation.[48] No other tumors have occurred in more than one patient to date except lipomas. However, we need to wait until larger numbers of people with Legius have been reported until possible associations with a low incidence can be confidently excluded. Messiaen et al.[44] estimate that to exclude rare complications with a prevalence of 1%, data from 250 well-characterized, preferably adult, patients are needed.

The majority of reported cases have been familial. The highest chance of finding a *SPRED1* mutation is in familial cases with ONLY NF1 pigmentary changes. In a cohort of sporadic patients with only CAL +/− freckling but no other NF1 mutations, Messiaen et al.[44] found a *SPRED1* mutation in 13/414 (1.3)%. However, in a familial cohort they detected 19% to have *SPRED1* mutations (18/94). In both cohorts they found more NF1 mutations (414/957, 44%, in sporadic group and 69/94, 73%, in familial group).

In terms of follow-up of Legius syndrome, given the association with learning problems, we currently follow children annually until the age of 7 years, but thereafter annual review seems unnecessary. In their most recent publication the Legius group suggests 3 yearly review.[46] However, the families should be asked to report unusual medical problems to exclude any association with the syndrome.

NF1 Exon 17 3-bp Inframe Deletion (c.2970_2972delAAT)

Upadhyaya et al.[42] reported 21 unrelated probands (14 familial and 7 sporadic) with the same c.2970–2972 del AAT (p.990delM) mutation but no cutaneous neurofibromas and no clinically obvious plexiform Neurofibromas. Of the total cohort (n = 47), only one had had a symptomatic spinal neurofibroma removed. Thirty of the forty-seven individuals had axillary freckling. There was a different frequency of complications, with a much lower frequency of learning problems, macrocephaly, and short stature; a similar frequency of scoliosis but with an increased frequency of pulmonary stenosis than in an ordinary NF1 cohort. The main importance of the phenotype was the lack of dermal neurofibromas in adult patients.

Since the initial publication, there has been one further report[17] of a child with NF1 pigmentary changes only. This child was identified when a cohort of 151 patients satisfying the NF1 diagnostic criteria, and followed in a primarily pediatric NF1 clinic, were tested initially for SPRED1 (2 patients identified) and then exon 17 sequenced in the reminder. In our own clinic we have found no further patients with the deletion when testing adults with CAL only. It is a less common cause of the CAL phenotype than *SPRED1* mutations.

Neuro-Cardio-Facial Cutaneous (NCFC) Syndromes and Their Overlap with NF1

Introduction

The overlap of clinical features, particularly in facial appearance, learning disability, short stature, macrocephaly (true and relative), and cardiac involvement, between NF1, Noonan, LEOPARD, cardio-facio-cutaneous (CFC), and Costello syndromes has been recognized for some years. There is also overlap in the kind of malignancies which can occur. The conditions have now been shown to be caused by mutations in genes in the same molecular pathway.[49,50] The RAS mitogen-activated protein kinase (RAS/MAPK) pathway has been most studied because of its critical role in cancer pathogenesis; the fact that the same genes cause these syndromes highlights their key role in developmental processes. It also raises the prospect that drugs developed to control the pathway in cancer may be effective in their treatment.

The two most common conditions, NF1 and Noonan syndrome are notable for their extreme variability, even within families. The identification of genes in the same pathway in this group of conditions with overlapping features raises the possibility that functional polymorphisms in different pathway genes affect the expression of causative mutations in others.

The term NCFC syndromes is used by some as a collective term for the group of conditions,[49] others simply refer to "RASopathies."[50] In this section there is a brief clinical description of each disorder. The key features and causative genes are summarized in Table 3.4 and the pathway itself is illustrated in Fig. 3.6. Inheritance in all is autosomal dominant. Other than NF1 and Noonan syndrome, the syndromes are rare.

In clinical practice, the only pathway syndrome that cannot be distinguished clinically from NF1 is Legius syndrome. Although CAL spots are reported as features of Noonan and LEOPARD syndrome, there are nearly always sufficient

TABLE 3.4. Summary of features of other neuro-cardio-facio-cutaneous syndromes which overlap with NF1 and Legius syndrome.

	Noonan	LEOPARD	Cardio-facio-cutaneous	Costello
Year of first description	1965	1969	1986	1977
Overlapping cutaneous features	Café au lait spots described more frequently than general population	CAL spots reported in 70–80% and usually precede lentigines; lentigines develop in skin-folds	CAL spots reported but not confirmed in recent survey of 61 individuals; multiple melanocytic nevi common	Although generalized increased pigmentation reported, CAL are not. Skin tends to be loose and soft, particularly on palms – possible overlap with NF1 microdeletion cases
Congenital heart disease	Pulmonary stenosis 20–50%	Pulmonary stenosis 25%	Pulmonary stenosis: frequency uncertain	Pulmonary stenosis in ~30%
Hypertrophic obstructive cardiomyopathy (HOCM) – if this is associated with NF1 at all is uncertain	20–30% presenting at birth or developing in childhood	Detected in up to 70% usually developing in infancy	HOCM: frequency uncertain	30–47% develop HOCM in infancy or early childhood
Psychomotor development	25% have learning problems and 10–15% require special education	Mild learning problems in approximately 30%	Majority have moderate to severe developmental problems	Mild to moderate developmental delay in all children

Associated tumors	Increased risk of Juvenile myelomonocytic and acute myeloid leukemias; also giant cell lesions (benign tumor-like lesions frequently affecting jaws but also other bones or soft tissues).	Individual case reports,[51] of myelodysplasia, acute myelogenous leukemia, neuroblastoma, malignant melanoma, and bilateral choristomas (a congenital corneal tumor)	Single cases: acute lymphoblastic leukemia, hepatoblastoma (patient immunosuppressed), non-Hodgkin lymphoma, and large B-cell lymphoma	Overall childhood tumor frequency 17%. Rhabdomyosarcoma most frequent tumor of early childhood followed by neuroblastoma; transitional cell carcinoma of bladder occurs in adolescents

Source: Data compiled from Burkitt Wright and Kerr,[49] Sarkozy et al,[51] Allanson,[52] Gelb and Tartaglia,[53] Rauen[54] and Gripp and Lin[55]

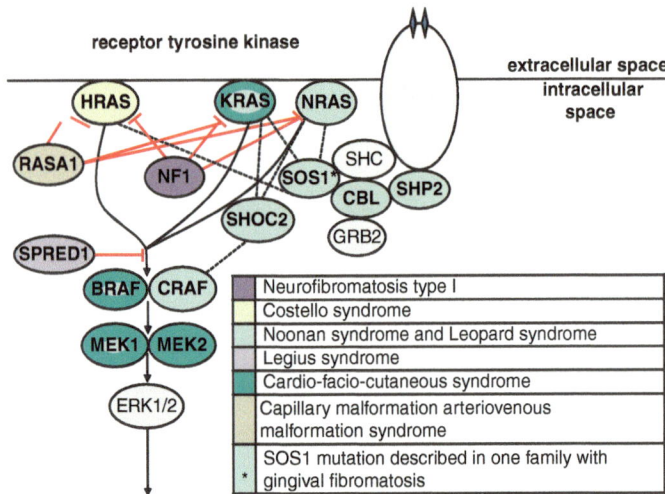

FIGURE 3.6. The RasMAPK pathway and associated syndromes.

distinguishing features from NF1 and skinfold freckling does not occur – although the lentigines in LEOPARD do involve the skin folds. The only condition I have seen misdiagnosed as NF1 is LEOPARD syndrome. The other syndromes have all been delineated much more recently than NF1 and it may be that more overlapping complications will emerge as adults with the different syndromes are followed. Given the underlying overlap in pathogenesis we need to be alert in the clinic for the occurrence of similar rare tumors or other problems. A good example of this is in Legius syndrome; there have been two cases reported with vascular anomalies, not something we would associate with NF1, but because of the association of mutations in RASA1 in capillary malformation–AV malformation syndrome, it becomes a possible true association.[10,44,50]

Noonan Syndrome

Noonan syndrome is at least as common as NF1.[52] The main clinical findings are short stature, pectus abnormalities, congenital heart defects (usually pulmonary stenosis and hypertrophic cardiomyopathy), learning disorders, and a characteristic facial appearance (ptosis, posteriorly rotated ears and hypertelorism). CAL spots are reported to occur more commonly in Noonan syndrome but no other overlapping skin features.

Is There a Neurofibromatosis Noonan Syndrome?

It has long been debated whether there is a specific syndrome which combines the features of NF1 and Noonan.[56,57] However, when cohorts of patients with NF1 have been systematically surveyed no evidence for a specific syndrome has emerged,[58] and this has always been my impression. Some people with NF1 had facial features which overlap with Noonan's but these did not routinely segregate in families.[58] The other overlapping features are pectus abnormalities and pulmonary stenosis. When mutation analysis has been done in cohorts of individuals with NF1 but Noonan-like facies mutations in the NF1 gene alone have been found.[59]

LEOPARD Syndrome

The name LEOPARD is an acronym for the common disease features: multiple **L**entigines, **E**lectrocardiographic conduction abnormalities, **O**cular hypertelorism, **P**ulmonary stenosis, **A**bnormal genitalia, **R**etardation of growth, and sensorineural **D**eafness.[51,53] In practice the overlap with NF1 mainly arises because of the lentigines and occasional CAL spots – the lentigines can develop in skin folds causing further confusion. In distinction from the freckles in NF1, the lentigines in LEOPARD are consistently darker and, in my experience, slightly raised above the skin (Fig. 3.7).

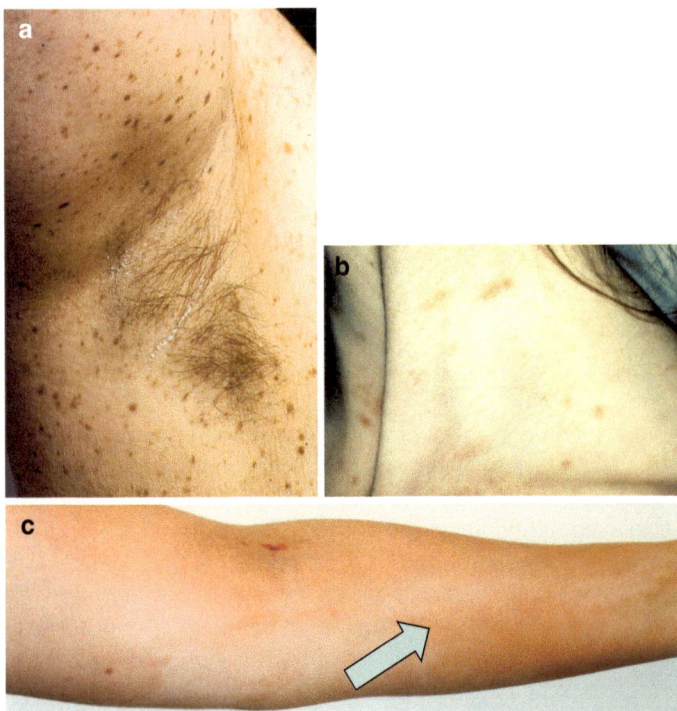

FIGURE 3.7. The differential diagnosis of NF1 skin lesions: (**a**) The lentigines in LEOPARD syndrome; note axillary involvement-patient originally diagnosed as NF1. (**b**) Urticaria pigmentosa: note the *orangey-brown* skin lesions with superficial resemblance to CAL spots; however, the lesions are slightly raised. (**c**) Fake tan giving impression of segmental CAL pigmentation.

Costello and Cardio-Facio-Cutaneous (CFC) Syndromes

These are the most severe of the RASopathies.[49,54,55] Affected children usually present in infancy with severe feeding problems and failure to thrive; nearly all cases are significantly developmentally delayed. As these are not usually seen in

NF1, the conditions are rarely confused. The other feature common in Costello and CFC, but not usually seen in other NCFC syndromes, is abnormal hair. The facies in both conditions may be relatively normal at birth but become coarse with age.

Costello Syndrome

Features which suggest Costello syndrome include neonatal atrial arrhythmias, excess skin which darkens with age, papillomas (usually after age 2 years), and ulnar deviation of the hands with deep palmar creases.[49,55] Approximately 15% of patients develop solid tumors particularly embryonic rhabdomyosarcomas, neuroblastomas, and bladder carcinoma (from teenage years onward).

CFC Syndrome

In CFC, more severe developmental problems and underlying brain abnormalities often predominate the clinical picture, with 50% of patients developing seizures which may present with infantile spasms.[49,54] Ectodermal abnormalities are also often a predominant feature with absent eyebrows (ulerythema ophryogenes) and keratosis pilaris. Whether there is a risk of associated malignancy remains to be established; there has been single cases of hepatoblastoma (in an immunosuppressed patient after cardiac transplantation), acute lymphoblastic leukemia, nonHodgkin's lymphoma, and large B cell lymphoma.

Other Pathway Disorders

The other two pathway disorders (Capillary malformation–AV malformation syndrome caused by mutations in *RASA1*, and the form of multiple hereditary gingivomatosis caused by mutation in *SOS1*) have no major overlapping features with NF1.

Constitutional Mismatch Repair Deficiency (CMMR-D): A Rare But Important Cause of a Phenotype Overlapping with NF1

This syndrome is rare but many of the reported cases were initially diagnosed as NF1 and it has therefore become an important condition to be aware of when assessing children with ?generalized/mosaic NF1. The syndrome is characterized by the development of childhood cancers, mainly hematological malignancies and/or brain tumors, as well as early onset colon cancers; some authors refer to CMMR-D as "Childhood cancer syndrome" or by the acronym (CoLoN), Colon tumors or/and leukemia/Lymphoma or/and Neurofibromatosis features.[60-63]

Inheritance is recessive and the syndrome is caused by biallelic mutations in one of four mismatch repair genes (*MLH1, MSH2, MSH6, PMS2*) – heterozygous mutations in the genes are associated with dominantly inherited nonpolyposis colon cancer (HNPCC). However, only approximately half the reported cases have a significant history of familial cancer. This is particularly the case for families with *PMS2* mutations probably related to the higher age of onset and reduced penetrance of heterozygous *PMS2*.

Wimmer and Kratz[61] recently reviewed the reported cases and added three more (*n*=92). These patients had had a total of 132 malignancies: 30 hematological (lymphoma/leukemia), 44 Brain Tumors (mainly glioblastoma and other astrocytic tumors), and 51 cases of HNPCC-associated cancers but with a much lower age of onset. There were single cases of neuroblastoma, Wilms tumor, rhabdomyosarcoma, ovarian neuroectodermal tumor, infantile myofibromatosis, breast cancer, and sarcoma.

The overlap with NF1 arises because 63/92 reported cases have café au lait macules. Some reports[63,64] have emphasized that the CAL in CMMR-D are atypical with irregular outlines and patchy pigmentation; areas of skin hypopigmentation are also reported. However, a proportion of the cases have other significant NF1 features including skin fold freckling, Lisch nodules, and pseudarthrosis and satisfy NIH diagnostic criteria. In addition, in some of the cases the skin changes were segmental in distribution suggesting a somatic NF1 mutation. One of the cases with CMMR-D due to homozygous MLH1 mutations has been shown to have an NF1 truncating mutation.[65] There is also evidence that the NF1 gene is a mutational target of MMR deficiency. It therefore seems that at least in some CMMR-D cases there has been somatic NF1 mutation giving rise to the children having the additional phenotype of generalized or segmental NF1.

Although rare, these cases are important to recognize because of the more severe cancer phenotype than normal NF1, the 25% recurrence risk for sibs, and the increased colon cancer risks in the heterozygous parents and their extended families.

When to Think About CMMR-D in a Child Presenting with Multiple CAL Spots or Segmental NF1

- Consanguinous parents
- Sibling or cousin (in consanguineous families) with childhood cancer
- If child has had one of the CMMR-D related malignancies – the majority of which would be unusual in ordinary NF1
- Family history of colon cancer or other HNPCC-associated tumors

CAL in Other Mismatch Repair Disorders

This group of conditions includes ataxia telangiectasia, Fanconi's anemia, Bloom syndrome, and Nijmegen break syndrome. They are all recessively inherited and usually the other presenting features mean that the differential of NF1 is never considered. They are not associated with typical CAL but can have multiple atypical lesions with irregular outlines and variable depth of pigmentation.[9]

NF1: Differential Diagnosis – Other Conditions

Introduction

The conditions which tend to get misdiagnosed as NF1 fall into three categories – those with pigmentary features that have CAL spots or patchy skin pigmentation, those with pigmentary features misdiagnosed as CAL, and those with tumors misdiagnosed as neurofibromas. A fourth, extremely rare group is tumor predisposition syndromes in which both CAL and tumors that can be mistaken for neurofibromas occur. The first two tend to present in childhood and the clinical clues come from assessing whether other problems the child has are typical for NF1 and in the assessment of the patches themselves. The conditions with other tumors tend to present in adults and here the lack of CAL spots in childhood or other common NF1 childhood problems, like learning disability, are usually the pointers in the history.

The two commonest misdiagnoses are through overinterpretation of variation of normal skin variation in childhood and lipomas in adults. The other conditions are all extremely rare and even in specialist practice I have only ever seen one or two cases of each – in all cases there were major clinical clues to the fact this could not be typical NF1. For this reason I have just given a brief description of each condition based on three main reference sources.[66-68] Shah[9] has recently reviewed the diagnostic and clinical significance of CAL spots and the syndromes with which they are strongly/weakly associated. I have only included conditions which I have seen personally, as I presume this means they are very rarely confused with NF1.

Conditions with CAL Spots and Other Patchy Skin Pigmentation Changes

Variation of Normal Skin Pigmentation

When I first started an NF clinic, this group of patients probably represented the one which caused me most confusion and the families' unnecessary concern. Over the years I have gradually learned about the different normal pigmentary patterns one sees in different ethnic groups. For example, in black skin I have seen children with marked pigmentation after scarring (e.g., after an insect bite or chicken pox); if they have one or two CAL as variation of normal and the pigmented scars are then counted, they can be mistakenly labeled as having NF1.

When we are assessing possible mosaic skin changes, then the clue are segments of skin with increased/decreased pigmentation often with well-demarcated borders. The other reason large areas of pigmentation are important in NF1 is they may be the first clue in early childhood to an area where a plexiform neurofibroma may develop; in this case there may also be excessive hair growth. However, there are some natural pigmentary demarcation boundaries that should not be confused. These lines are often more obvious in darkly skinned individuals – the one that has most often caught my attention in the ?NF1 setting is the line which runs down the anterolateral line in the upper arm.[68] The other thing that has caught me out has been use of artificial tanning – the patients having to point out to me the cause of their apparently "affected" segment (Fig. 3.7)!

The final group in this category is that which my NF mentor, Professor Vic Riccardi, refers to as "Pigmentary miscegeny." These are the skin changes seen when children have parents with very different skin coloring, usually from different ethnic groups but also if one parent has very pale skin and the other very dark. These children can have a mixture of hypo- and hyperpigmented patches – the latter tend to have very irregular outlines and depth of pigmentation. In our own clinic we see several children a year referred as ?NF1 where this is the cause. If the children have any other problems, one needs to ensure there is not an alternative diagnosis which might produce pigmentation with irregular depth/outline such as the DNA repair disorders.

Rare Disorders with Typical CAL Spots

These are the two disorders where I have seen cases with absolutely typical NF1-like CAL spots. In both the other problems the children had were not typical for NF1 and the distinction from NF1 had already been made when I reviewed them. Typical CAL are also reported in Russell Silver syndrome.

1. *Ring chromosome syndromes*: Ring chromosomes occur when part of one end of the chromosome is deleted and the two ends then "stick" together. Problems occur as the ring structure is unstable in mitosis. CAL spots have been reported in a variety of ring chromosome cases (chromosomes 7, 11, 12, 15 and 17[9]). The other clues to diagnosis are usually more profound development problems than in NF1, shorter stature, microcephaly, and dysmorphic facial features.
2. *Schimke immunoosseus dysplasia*: This is an autosomal recessive condition characterized by growth retardation, renal failure, recurrent infections, cerebral infarcts, and skin pigmentation beginning in childhood. The majority of cases are caused by mutations in the *SMARCAL1* gene. I have only seen one case but the skin changes were typical NF1-like CAL with skin fold freckling.

McCune Albright Syndrome

The major features of this disorder are polyostotic fibrous dysplasia, precocious puberty and other endocrinopathies, and large, segmental areas of CAL pigmentation. It is sporadic and caused by postzygotic mutations in the *GNAS1* gene.

The distinction from NF1 is usually straightforward as the areas of CAL are much larger than normal with no associated smaller CAL. They also tend to follow the lines of Blaschko.[68] The CAL in McCune Albright characteristically have a jagged outline said to resemble "the coast of Maine" compared with the smooth contours in NF1 a likened to the "coast of California." This is however, not universal as sometimes the large CAL overlying plexiforms can have a jagged edge (Fig. 3.2). The more reliable diagnostic aids are the presence of multiple much smaller lesions in NF1 and the other features in McCune Albright.

Conditions with Skin Lesions Misdiagnosed as CAL Spots

Urticaria Pigmentosa

This is the most common variant of childhood mastocytosis. The skin lesions usually develop in the first year of life, are slightly elevated, and their color can be brown–red or yellow. As they develop the lesions, when brown can be confused with CAL (Fig. 3.7). However, as they develop they become either plaque-like or popular and this distinguishes them from CAL. The clue to etiology is elicited by "Darier's sign": when a lesion is scratched a marked urticarial reaction is usually elicited.

Congenital Melanocytic Nevi

When congenital melanocytic nevi are particularly large and cover a major part of the body (e.g., bathing trunk distribution), they can be confused with the skin changes seen over some plexiform neurofibromas. Both may first appear as just flat pigmented lesions, and then the lesion becomes thickened with time – in the case of NF1 with plexiform change histologically. The congenital nevi are usually much darker than NF1-associated CAL and carry a risk of melanomatous change not seen in NF1.

Conditions with Tumors

Multiple Lipomatosis

Multiple lipomas are the "commonest" misdiagnosis we see in adults in NF1, even this accounts for only a handful of cases a year at most. Inheritance is autosomal dominant and my impression is that penetrance may not be 100%. The lipomas present as subcutaneous swellings, which are usually painless (in contrast to peripheral nerve neurofibromas/ schwannomas), and usually grow to several centimeters in diameter or larger. They tend to cluster on the forearms, thighs, lower chest wall, and abdomen. The distinction from nerve tumors is the lack of pain and they are usually softer on palpation. The other major distinction from NF1 is the lack of associated pigmentary changes.

Steatocystoma Multiplex

This is a rare dominant disorder caused by mutations in the keratin 17 gene. Affected individuals develop painful cutaneous swellings, arising from the sweat glands, from childhood onward (Fig. 3.7). The lesions have a yellowish color and firm consistency which on biopsy show disordered sebaceous gland elements.

Proteus Syndrome

The most famous misdiagnosis of NF1 historically was the Elephant man, Joseph Merrick. In 1986, Tibbles and Cohen[69] suggested the alternative diagnosis of Proteus syndrome and this is now widely accepted. Proteus is an extremely rare disorder characterized by asymmetrical overgrowth of almost any part of the body, associated with epidermal and connective tissue nevi, dysregulated growth of fatty tissue (lipomas or regional absence), bony hyperostosis, and vascular malformations.

The overlap with NF1 is because some of the overgrown areas can resemble plexiform neurofibromas. I have seen two cases where plexiform neurofibromas affecting the feet were initially thought to represent the connective tissue nevi of Proteus, with the "moccasin sole" appearance. The distinguishing feature clinically is that the plexiforms are usually soft in consistency whereas the connective tissue nevi in Proteus are firm on palpation.

Rare Autosomal Dominant Tumor Predisposition Syndromes

This group is summarized in Table 3.5. In my experience they are easily distinguishable from NF1 clinically. However, as both CAL and cutaneous lesions which can be mistakenly labeled as neurofibromas occur I have included them. The important thing is to remember them when assessing patients that "don't fit" for NF1.

NF1 Diagnostic Criteria: Pitfalls

The NIH NF1 diagnostic criteria agreed at a 1987 consensus meeting[70] are:

The clinical diagnosis is made when at least two of the following are present:

- A first-degree relative with NF1
- Six or more café au lait patches >0.5 cm in children and >1.5 cm in adults
- Axillary or groin freckling
- Two or more neurofibromas of any type or one plexiform neurofibroma
- Two or more Lisch nodules (iris hamartomas)
- Optic pathway glioma
- Bony dysplasia of the sphenoid wing
- Thinning of the long bone cortex with or without pseudarthrosis of the long bones

TABLE 3.5. Rare dominant tumor predisposition syndromes where a diagnosis of a form of NF may initially be considered.

Name	Key features	Overlap with neurofibromatosis
PTEN hamartoma tumor syndrome (includes Cowden syndrome, Banayan–Ruvalcaba–Riley Syndrome (BRRS))	Cowden phenotype: a multiple hamartoma syndrome, high risk of benign and malignant tumors of the thyroid, breast, and endometrium. Affected individuals usually have macrocephaly, trichilemmomas, and papillomatous papules and present by the late 20s	CAL spots reported
	BRRS is a congenital disorder characterized by macrocephaly, intestinal hamartomatous polyposis, lipomas, and pigmented macules of the glans penis; up to 50% have developmental/learning problems	Misdiagnosis of skin or GI lesions (ganglioneuromas can occur)
	PTEN mutations found in some individuals presenting with autistic spectrum and macrocephaly	Macrocephaly: in PTEN syndromes head circumference nearly always ≥ 97th centile, whereas in NF1 may just be relative macrocephaly

Carney complex Has also been referred to by two acronyms: NAME – nevi, atrial myxomas, ephelides and LAMB – lentigines, atrial myxoma, blue nevi	Pale brown to black lentingines: develop in increasing numbers from early childhood, occur anywhere, particularly affect face around the eyes, nose, and mouth Myxomas: cutaneous, cardiac, and breast predominantly Endocrine tumors: including primary pigmentary nodular adrenocortical disease, testicular tumors, and thyroid adenomas Psammomatous melanotic schwannoma (PMS): PMS may occur anywhere in the central and peripheral nervous system; it is most frequently found in the nerves of the gastrointestinal tract (esophagus and stomach) and paraspinal sympathetic chain	CAL spots reported Skin myxomas misdiagnosed as neurofibromas PMS pathology very specific but presentation could be same as a lesion in NF1/NF2
Multiple endocrine neoplasia syndrome type one and 2B	MEN1 associated with parathyroid adenoma, pituitary adenoma, pancreatic islet cell adenoma, lipoma, gingival papules, facial angiofibromas, collagenomas MEN2B associated with mucosal neuromas, pheochromocytoma, medullary thyroid cancer, parathyroid adenoma, and marfanoid habitus	CAL spots reported in both Mucosal neuromas misdiagnosed as neurofibromas in MEN2B Pheochromocytoma in MEN2B

In the majority of cases the diagnosis of NF1 is straight-forward and the NIH diagnostic criteria have stood the test of time well until recently. However, caution now needs to be made because the recognition of Legius syndrome and CMMR-D as follows:

1. Individuals with CAL and axillary freckling but nothing else may have Legius syndrome, particularly if there is a family history of the same phenotype.
2. The term first-degree relative includes parents, children, and siblings. As CMMR-D is autosomal recessive they could be diagnosed with NF1 on the grounds of CAL spots and an affected sibling and the much more serious diagnosis, with a different inheritance pattern, missed.
3. It is possible for people with segmental NF1 to have ≥6 CAL and unilateral skinfold freckling in an affected segment BUT they do not have generalized NF1 and the importance of the distinction is the lower frequency of complications and offspring recurrence risk.

NF1 Genetic Testing Indications

The fact that the clinical diagnosis is usually straightforward, combined with little demand for prenatal testing, the large gene size, and lack of recurrent mutations all contributed to little use of NF1 gene testing in routine clinical practice until relatively recently. With improved mutation detection (95% using most complete methods[3]), the recognition of clinically useful genotype–phenotypes, and Legius syndrome this is now changing.

At the current time our clinic testing criteria are:

1. Those who may have deletions on clinical grounds
2. Those with an atypical phenotype for diagnostic clarification
3. Families with two or more generations with isolated pigmentary changes (*NF1* and *SPRED1*)
4. Children with no family history and isolated pigmentary changes (*NF1* and *SPRED1*)
5. Someone considering prenatal/preimplantation diagnosis

NF2: Differential Diagnosis and Related Conditions

Introduction

Had NF1 and NF2 not been historically lumped together as one disease, it would be more appropriate for NF2 and the related disorder schwannomatosis to be classified as different types of "schwannomatoses." With improved imaging techniques and molecular testing the diagnosis of NF2 is usually straightforward and there are a very limited number of true differentials. In both schwannomatosis and multiple meningiomas the diagnosis can only be made after exclusion of NF2.

Schwannomatosis

Patients with schwannomatosis develop peripheral nerve and spinal root schwannomas almost exclusively, but with no skin tumors. Cranial nerve involvement is rare. There is no eye involvement, ependymomas have not been seen, and meningiomas occur very rarely.[71-73] The appearance of the tumors is clinically and radiologically the same as in NF2. However, the tumors in schwannomatosis are usually associated with more persistent pain than just the transient paraesthesia in response to pressure that most peripheral nerve lesions cause. The problem is that if a sporadic patient presents with peripheral and/or spinal lesions there is no way of knowing if this is mosaic NF2 or schwannomatosis. Diagnostic criteria for Schwannomatosis have been proposed[73] (Table 3.6). Patient assessment includes a thorough cutaneous and eye examination for signs of NF2, full MRI neuroaxis imaging, and NF2 mutation testing.

The majority of cases of schwannomatosis are sporadic. The risk to offspring of sporadic cases is much less than 50%. In familial cases inheritance is dominant but expression is variable and incomplete penetrance is recorded.[73] Some patients present with multiple lesions localized to one body part suggesting a mosaic genetic mechanism; whether it is mosaic NF2 or Schwannomatosis can only be evaluated by molecular analysis in tumors.

TABLE 3.6. Diagnostic criteria for schwannomatosis proposed by MacCollin et al.[73]

Definite schwannomatosis
- Age >30 years AND
- ≥2 nonintradermal schwannomas, at least one with histologic confirmation AND no evidence of vestibular tumor on high-quality MRI scan AND no known constitutional NF2 mutation

OR

- One pathologically confirmed nonvestibular schwannoma plus a first-degree relative who meets above criteria

Possible schwannomatosis
- Age <30 AND
- ≥2 nonintradermal schwannomas, at least one with histologic confirmation AND no evidence of vestibular tumor on high-quality MRI scan AND no known constitutional NF2 mutation

OR

- Age >45 years AND ≥2 nonintradermal schwannomas, at least one with histologic confirmation AND no symptoms of 8th nerve dysfunction AND no known constitutional NF2 mutation

OR

- Radiographic evidence of a nonvestibular schwannoma and first-degree relative meeting criteria for definite schwannomatosis

Segmental schwannomatosis
- Meets criteria for definite or possible but limited to one limb or ≤5 contiguous segments of spine

The genetic mechanisms underlying schwannomatosis are gradually being elucidated. The gene has been localized to chromosome 22 proximal to NF2 and mutations in the SMARCB1 tumor suppressor gene reported in 2007.[74] Subsequent reports suggest that between 33 and 66% of familial cases[75,76] and 7%[75] of sporadic cases have germline SMARCB1 mutations. Mutations in the same gene also cause inherited predisposition to rhabdoid tumors, the tumors developing after a somatic "second hit." The major question is therefore why are the two phenotypes so different? Tumor analysis has shown a complex mechanism of tumorigenesis in schwannomatosis which requires somatic mutation in both copies of the *NF2* gene as well as in *INI1*.[75,77] Two families with both meningiomas and schwannomas with SMARCB1 mutations have also been reported.[78,79]

In the clinical setting tumor analysis can be used to determine if a sporadic case, with normal lymphocyte mutation testing for *NF2* and *SMARCB1* represents mosaic NF2 or schwannomatosis. In mosaic NF2 each separate tumor will share one mutation in common, whereas in schwannomatosis the *NF2* mutations are different in each tumor.

Multiple Meningiomas

Multiple meningiomas can occur as part of NF2 or as a separate genetic entity dominant inheritance of multiple meningiomas and no other features; this is a very rare entity. Linkage to NF2 was excluded in one family and other genes have not yet been identified.[80] As for schwannomatosis, the diagnosis of familial non-NF2 meningiomas can only be made with a clear family history. In sporadic cases, the causes include NF2 mosaicism, or noncontiguous spread of a single sporadic tumor or new mutation in the as yet unidentified gene(s) responsible for non-NF2 familial meningiomas.

The clinical approach to the patient with multiple meningiomas is like that for schwannomas; NF2 must be excluded initially.

Misdiagnosis of Other Cerebello-Pontine (CP) Angle Tumors as Vestibular Schwannomas

This is an extremely rare event but most NF2 clinics have had one or two cases referred where other tumors in the CP angle are initially diagnosed as vestibular schwannomas. These have included choroid plexus papillomas (which can further mimic NF2 by seeding down the spine) and lymphoma.[81]

Acknowledgments   I am grateful to Dr. Rick Whitehouse for providing Fig. 3.5, Dr. Emma Burkitt Wright for Fig. 3.6, and to the patients who have allowed me to use their pictures and clinical histories.

References

1. Huson SM, Harper PS, Compston DAS. Von Recklinghausen neurofibromatosis: a clinical and population study in South East Wales. *Brain*. 1988;111:1355-1382.
2. Friedman JM, Birch PH. Type one neurofibromatosis: a descriptive analysis of the disorder in 1728 patients. *Am J Med Genet*. 1997;70: 138-143.
3. Messiaen LM, Callens T, Mortier G, et al. Exhaustive mutation analysis of the NF1 gene allows identification of 95% of mutations and reveals a high frequency of unusual splicing defects. *Hum Mutat*. 2000;15(6):541.
4. Kehrer-Sawatski H, Coopper DN. Mosaicism in sporadic neurofibromatosis type one: Variations on a theme common to other hereditary cancer syndromes? *J Med Genet*. 2008;45:622-631.
5. Moyhuddin A, Baser ME, Watson C, et al. Somatic mosaicism in neurofibromatosis 2: prevalence and risk of disease transmission to offspring. *J Med Genet*. 2003;40:459-463.
6. Huson SM, Korf BR. The phakomatoses. In: Rimoin DL, Connor JM, Pyeritz RE, Korf BR, eds. *Principles and Practice of Medical Genetics*. 5th ed. Edinburgh: Churchill Livingstone; 2006.
7. Rahman N, Scott R. Cancer genes associated with phenotypes in monallelic and biallelic mutation carriers: new lessons from old players. *Hum Mol Genet*. 2007;16(special no 1):R60-R68.
8. Ragge NK. Clinical and genetic patterns of neurofibromatosis 1 and 2. *Br J Ophthalmol*. 1993;77(10):662-672.
9. Shah KN. The diagnostic and clinical significance of café-au-lait macules. *Pediatr Clin N Am*. 2010;57:1131-1153.
10. Spurlock G, Bennett E, Chuzhanova N, et al. SPRED1 mutations (Legius syndrome): another clinically useful genotype for dissecting the neurofibromatosis type one phenotype. *J Med Genet*. 2009;46: 431-437.
11. Evans DGR, Huson SM, Donnai D, et al. A clinical study of type 2 neurofibromatosis. *Q J Med*. 2010;304:603-618.
12. Ruggieri M, Huson SM. The clinical and diagnostic implications of mosaicism in the neurofibromatoses. *Neurology*. 2001;56:1433-1434.
13. Maertens O, Schepper SD, Vandesompele J, et al. Molecular dissection of isolated disease features in mosaic neurofibromatosis type one. *Am J Hum Genet*. 2007;81:243-251.

14. Evans DGR, Wallace A, Truman L, Strachan T. Mosaicism in classical neurofibromatosis type two: A common mechanism for sporadic disease in tumor prone syndromes? *Am J Hum Genet*. 1998;63: 727-736.
15. Huson SM, Clark D, Compston DAS, Harper PS. A genetic study of von Recklinghausen neurofibromatosis in South East Wales I: prevalence, fitness, mutation rate and effect of parental transmission on severity. *J Med Genet*. 1989;26:704-711.
16. Messiaen L, Vogt J, Bengesser K, et al. Mosaic type-1 NF1 microdeletions as a cause of both generalised and segmental neurofibromatosis type one. *Hum Mutat*. 2010;Nov 30. Epub ahead of print.
17. Muram-Zborovski TM, Vaughn CP, Viskochil DH. NF1 exon 22 analysis of individuals with the clinical diagnosis of neurofibromatosis type 1. *Am J Med Genet*. 2010;152A(pt A):1973-1978.
18. Pasmant E, Sabbagh A, Spurlock G, et al. NF1 microdeletions in neurofibromatosis type one: from genotype to phenotype. *Hum Mutat Mutat Brief*. 2010;31:E1506-E1516.
19. Mautner VF, Kluwe L, Friedrich RE. Clinical characterisation of 29 neurofibromatosis type one patients with molecularly ascertained 1.4 Mb type one NF1 deletions. *J Med Genet*. 2010;47(9):623-630.
20. Tinschert S. Clinical phenotypes in patients with *NF1* microdeletions. In: Kaufmann D, ed. *Neurofibromatoses, Monographs in Human Genetics 16*. Basel: S. Karger; 2008:78-88.
21. Venturin M, Guarnieri P, Natacci F. Mental retardation and cardiovascular malformation in NF1 microdeleted patients point to candidate genes in 17q11.2. *J Med Genet*. 2004;41:35-41.
22. Mensink KA, Ketterling RP, Flynn HC, et al. Connective tissue dysplasia in five new patients with NF1 microdeletions: further expansion of phenotype and review of the literature. *J Med Genet*. 2006;43:e08.
23. De Raedt T, Brems H, Wolkenstein P, et al. Elevated risk for MPNST in NF1 microdeletion patients. *Am J Hum Genet*. 2003;72: 1288-1292.
24. Descheemaeker MJ, Roelandts K, De Raedt T, et al. Intelligence in individuals with a neurofibromatosis type 1 microdeletion. *Am J Med Genet A*. 2004;131:325-326.
25. Spiegel M, Oexle K, Horn D, et al. Childhood overgrowth in patients with common NF1 microdeletions. *Eur J Hum Genet*. 2005;13: 883e8.
26. Korf BR, Schneider G, Poussaint TY. Structural anomalies revealed by neuroimaging studies in the brains of patients with neurofibromatosis type 1 and large deletions. *Genet Med*. 1999;1:136e40.
27. Douglas J, Cilliers D, Coleman K, et al. Mutations in RNF135, a gene within the NF1 microdeletion region, cause phenotypic abnormalities including overgrowth. *Nat Genet*. 2007;39:963-965.

28. Pulst SM, Riccardi VM, Fain P, Korenberg JR. Familial spinal neuro-fibromatosis: clinical and DNA linkage analysis. *Neurology*. 1991;41:1923-1925.
29. Poyhonen M, Leisti EL, Kytölä S, Leisti J. Hereditary spinal neurofi-bromatosis: A rare form of NF1? *J Med Genet*. 1997;34:184-187.
30. Ars E, Kruyer H, Gaona A, et al. A clinical variant of neurofibroma-tosis type 1: familial spinal neurofibromatosis with a frameshift mutation in the NF1 gene. *Am J Hum Genet*. 1998;62:834-841.
31. Kaufmann D, Müller R, Bartelt B, et al. Spinal neurofibromatosis without café-au-lait macules in two families with null mutations of the NF1 gene. *Am J Hum Genet*. 2001;69:1395-1400.
32. Kluwe L, Tatagiba M, Fünsterer C, Mautner VF. NF1 mutations and clinical spectrum in patients with spinal neurofibromas. *J Med Genet*. 2003;40(5):368-371.
33. Fauth C, Kehrer-Sawatski H, Zatkova A, et al. Two sporadic spinal neurofibromatosis patients with malignant peripheral nerve sheath tumour. *Eur J Hum Genet*. 2009;52:409-414.
34. Messiaen L, Riccardi V, Peltonen J, et al. Independent NF1 muta-tions in two large families with spinal neurofibromatosis. *J Med Genet*. 2003;40:122-126.
35. Messiaen L, Callens T, Williams JB, et al. Genotype-phenotype cor-relations in spinal NF [abstract 985]. Presented at: Annual Meeting of The American Society of Human Genetics; October 25, 2007; San Diego, California. Available from: http://www.ashg.org/genetics/ashg07s/index.shtml.
36. Upadhyaya M, Spurlock G, Kluwe L. The spectrum of somatic and germline NF1 mutations in NF1 patients with spinal neurofibromas. *Neurogenetics*. 2009;10:251-263.
37. Watson GH. Pulmonary stenosis, cafè au lait spots, and dull intelli-gence. *Arch Dis Child*. 1967;42:303-307.
38. Allanson JE, Upadhyaya M, Watson GH, et al. Watson syndrome: Is it a subtype of type 1 neurofibromatosis? *J Med Genet*. 1991;28(11):752-756.
39. Tassabehji M, Strachan T, Sharland M, et al. Tandem duplication within a neurofibromatosis type I (NF1) gene exon in a family with features of Watson syndrome and Noonan syndrome. *Am J Hum Genet*. 1993;53:90.
40. Upadhyaya M, Shen M, Cherryson A, et al. Analysis of mutations at the neurofibromatosis 1 (NF1) locus. *Hum Mol Genet*. 1992;1(9):735-740.
41. Riccardi VM. The pathophysiology of neurofibromatosis: IV. Dermatological insights into heterogeneity and pathogenesis. *J Am Acad Dermatol*. 1980;3:157-166.
42. Upadhyaya M, Huson SM, Davies M, et al. A complete absence of cutaneous neurofibromas associated with a 3-bp in-frame deletion in exon 17 of the NF1 gene (c.2970_2972 delAAT): A clinically significant genotype-phenotype correlation? *Am J Hum Genet*. 2007;80:140-145.

43. Brems H, Chmara M, Sahbatou M, et al. Mutations in the SPRED1 gene cause a neurofibromatosis type 1-like phenotype. *Nat Genet.* 2007;29:1120-1126.
44. Messiaen L, Yao S, Brems H, et al. Clinical and mutational spectrum of neurofibromatosis type 1 – like syndrome. *JAMA.* 2009;302:2111-2118.
45. Pasmant E, Sabbagh A, Hanna N, et al. SPRED1 germline mutations cause a neurofibromatosis type 1 overlapping phenotype. *J Med Genet.* 2009;46:425-430.
46. Denayer E, Chmara M, Brems H, et al. Legius syndrome in fourteen families. *Hum Mutat Mutat Brief.* 2010;32:E1985-E1998.
47. Muram-Zborovski TM, Stevenson DA, Viskochil DH, et al. SPRED1 mutations in a neurofibromatosis clinic. *J Child Neurol.* 2010;25:1203-1209.
48. Lane KA, Anninger WV, Katowitz JA. Expanding the phenotype of a neurofibromatosis type 1-like syndrome: a patient with SPRED1 mutation and orbital manifestations: retraction. *Ophthal Plast Reconstr Surg.* 2010;26(2):145.
49. Burkitt Wright EMM, Kerr B. RAS-MAPK pathway disorders: important causes of congenital heart disease, feeding difficulties, developmental delay and short stature. *Arch Dis Child.* 2010;95:724-730.
50. Tidyman WE, Rauen KA. The RASopathies: developmental syndromes of Ras/MAPK pathway dysregulation. *Curr Opin Genet Dev.* 2009;19:230-236.
51. Sarkozy A, Diligilio MC, Dallapiccola B. LEOPARD syndrome. *Orphanet J Rare Dis.* 2008;3:13.
52. Allanson JE. Noonan syndrome. In: Pagon RA, Bird TD, Dolan CR, eds. *GeneReviews [Internet].* Seattle, WA: University of Washington; 1993.
53. Gelb BD, Tartaglia M. LEOPARD syndrome. In: Pagon RA, Bird TD, Dolan CR, eds. *GeneReviews [Internet].* Seattle, WA: University of Washington; 1993.
54. Rauen K. Cardiofaciocutanous syndrome. In: Pagon RA, Bird TD, Dolan CR, eds. *GeneReviews [Internet].* Seattle, WA: University of Washington; 1993.
55. Gripp KW, Lin AE. Costello syndrome. In: Pagon RA, Bird TD, Dolan CR, eds. *GeneReviews [Internet].* Seattle, WA: University of Washington; 1993.
56. Opitz JM, Weaver DD. The neurofibromatosis—Noonan syndrome. *Am J Med Genet.* 1985;21(3):477-490.
57. Stevenson DA, Swenson JJ, Viskochil DH. Neurofibromatosis type one and other syndromes in the Ras pathway. In: Kaufmann D, ed. *Neurofibromatoses, Monographs in Human Genetics 16.* Basel: S. Karger; 2008:32-45.
58. Colley A, Donnai D, Evans DG. Neurofibromatosis/Noonan phenotype: a variable feature of type 1 neurofibromatosis. *Clin Genet.* 1996;49(2):59.

59. Baralle D, Mattocks C, Kalidas K, et al. Different mutations in the NF1 gene are associated with Neurofibromatosis-Noonan syndrome (NFNS). *Am J Med Genet.* 2003;119A(1):1.
60. Wimmer K, Etzler J. Constitutional mismatch repair-deficiency syndrome: Have we so far seen only the tip of an iceberg? *Hum Genet.* 2008;124:105-122.
61. Wimmer K, Kratz CP. Constitutional mismatch repair-deficiency syndrome. *Haematologica.* 2010;95:699-701.
62. Bandipalliam P. Syndrome of early onset colon cancers, hematologic malignancies and features of neurofibromatosis in HNPCC families with homozygous mismatch repair mutations. *Familial Cancers.* 2005;4:323-333.
63. De Vos M, Hayward BE, Charlton R. PMS2 mutations in childhood cancer. *J Natl Cancer Inst.* 2006;98:358-361.
64. Scott RH, Mansour S, Pritchard-Jones K. Medulloblastoma, acute myelocytic leukemia and colonic carcinomas in a child with biallelic *MSH6* mutations. *Nat Clin Pract Oncol.* 2007;4(2):130-134.
65. Alotaibi H, Riccarione MD, Ozturk M. Homozygosity at variant MLH1 can lead to secondary mutations in NF1, neurofibromatosis type one and early onset leukemia. *Mutat Res.* 2008;637:209-214.
66. Pagon RA, Bird TD, Dolan CR, et al., eds. *GeneReviews [Internet].* Seattle, WA: University of Washington; 1993.
67. Online Mendelian Inheritance in Man, OMIM (TM). McKusick-Nathans Institute of Genetic Medicine, Johns Hopkins University (Baltimore,MD) and National Center for Biotechnology Information, National Library of Medicine (Bethesda, MD), 2011. http://www.ncbi.nlm.nih.gov/omim/.
68. Harper J, Oranje A, Prose N, eds. *Textbook of Pediatric Dermatology.* London: Blackwell Publishing; 2006.
69. Tibbles JAR, Cohen MM Jr. Proteus syndrome: the Elephant man diagnosed. *Br Med J.* 1986;293:683-685.
70. Stumpf D. Consensus development conference of neurofibromatosis. *Arch Neurol.* 1988;45:575-578.
71. Evans DGR, Mason S, Huson SM, Ponder M, Harding AE, Strachan T. Spinal and cutaneous schwannomatosis is a variant form of type 2 neurofibromatosis: a clinical and molecular study. *J Neurol Neurosurg Psychiatry.* 1997;62(4):361.
72. MacCollin M, Woodfin W, Kronn D, Short MP. Schwannomatosis: a clinical and pathological study. *Neurology.* 1996;46:1072-1079.
73. MacCollin M, Chiocca EA, Evans DG, et al. Diagnostic criteria for schwannomatosis. *Neurology.* 2005;64(11):1838.
74. Hulsebos TJM, Plomp AS, Wolterman RA, Robanus-Maandag EC, Baas F, Wesseling P. Germline mutation of INI1/SMARCB1 in familial schwannomatosis. *Am J Hum Genet.* 2007;80:805-810.

75. Hadfield KD, Newman WG, Bowers NL, et al. Molecular characterization of *SMARCB1* and *NF2* in familial and sporadic schwannomatosis. *J Med Genet*. 2008;45:332-339.
76. Boyd C, Smith MJ, Kluwe L, et al. Alterations in the *SMARCB1 (INI1)* tumor suppressor gene in familial schwannomatosis. *Clin Genet*. 2008;74:358-366.
77. Sestini R, Bacci C, Provenzano A, Genuardi M, Papi L. Evidence of a four-hit mechanism involving *SMARCB1* and *NF2* in schwannomatosis. *Hum Mutat*. 2008;29:227-231.
78. Bacci C, Sestina R, Provenzano A, et al. Schwannomatosis associated with multiple meningiomas due to a familial *SMARCB1* mutation. *Neurogenetics*. 2010;11:73-80.
79. . Christiaans I, Kenter SB, Brink HC, et al. Germline SMARCB1 mutation and somatic NF2 mutations in familial multiple meningiomas. *J Med Genet*. doi:10.1136/jmg.2010.082420.
80. Shen Y, Nunes F, Stemmer-Rachamimov A, et al. Genomic profiling distinguishes familial multiple and sporadic multiple meningiomas. *BMC Med Genomics*. 2009;2:42.
81. Bonneville F, Savatovsky J, Chiras J. Imaging of cerebellopontine angle lesions: an update, part 2: intra-axial lesions, skull base lesions that may invade the cPA region and non-enhancing extra-axial lesions. *Eur Radiol*. 2007;17(11):2908-2920.

Chapter 4
Psychological Impact
of the Neurofibromatoses

Rosalie E. Ferner

Quality of life involves all aspects that affect the
individual's life
    At a particular time point, quality of life assesses the
disparity between the individual's expectations and his
or her actual life experience.[1]

Neurofibromatosis 1 and 2 are inherited tumor suppressor conditions that cause lifelong medical problems and carry a large
psychological burden. Anxiety and depression are common but
unwelcome bedfellows. The formation of specialist neurofibromatosis clinics has highlighted the value of long-term psychological support both within the clinic setting and in the
community for people with NF1 and NF2 and their families.
Moreover, the advent of clinical therapeutic trials has focused
attention on developing objective measurements of quality of
life that are comparable in different medical institutions.

Neurofibromatosis 1

Unpredictability of Disease Complications

Neurofibromatosis 1 is the source of psychological distress
because of the unpredictability of the medical complications and
the worry of not knowing what to expect in terms of physical

R.E. Ferner et al., *Neurofibromatoses in Clinical Practice*,
DOI: 10.1007/978-0-85729-629-0_4,
© Springer-Verlag London Limited 2011

problems. There is a nagging wariness that minor symptoms may herald progressive disease and stress arises from a lifelong need to be vigilant about possible medical complications.

Need for Expert Clinicians

Many patients express disappointment at being fobbed off by clinicians who do not understand the disease and who attribute all medical complaints to neurofibromatosis 1. They may have difficulty in communicating their needs to the doctors if they are anxious or have learning difficulties.

"Doctors should not be so fast to relate all unexplained symptoms to NF1. Please examine people carefully and carry out tests when necessary. Please also bear in mind that some people with NF may not be able to describe their symptoms" (personal communication from Mr. David Edgerton who attends the Guy's and St. Thomas' NHS Foundation Trust (GSTT) Complex NF1 clinic).

There is a requirement from childhood onward to build up and maintain a relationship of trust with multiple clinicians and nurses and to attend regular clinics. As a result, children miss lessons, young people are unable to participate in social activities enjoyed by their peers, and adults in employment frequently use up annual leave in order to attend medical appointments. Although many patients embrace the idea of educating students and doctors about neurofibromatosis, they stress the need for sensitivity on the part of the clinician in interpreting the individual's wishes.

"A diagnosis of Neurofibromatosis meant that I spent more time attending outpatient hospital appointments than with my contemporaries, but I used to look forward to them. An appointment with my consultant was akin to seeing a family friend, a favourite uncle" (personal communication from Aoife Quinn, who attends GSTT Complex NF1 clinic).

"I was diagnosed with NF1 when I was five years old. The endless hospital check-ups were more of an adventure to start with, a day off school, a trip to London on the train with my mum, and as my father worked in London I was guaranteed a good lunch! This soon wore off as I grew older; why all the interest in me? All these people wanting to look and examine me, poke and prod at some of my lumps and look at some of the cafe au lait patches, that at that time I thought that everyone had" (personal communication from Mr. Jeremy Meechan who attends GSTT NF1 clinic).

Disfigurement

In ancient times the physical form of the body was regarded as an indicator of a person's character and worth in society. Physical beauty reflected moral harmony and intelligence, while an unattractive appearance signified unworthiness – a viewpoint that is untenable in twenty-first century society, but which influenced artists like Leonardo Da Vinci.[2]

Facial Plexiform Neurofibromas

Disfiguring neurofibromas of the face are uncommon in NF1 but have a deleterious effect on quality of life as children are ostracized by class mates and adults feel socially isolated and reluctant to leave home or to meet unfamiliar people. The recent success of a partial facial transplantation for an individual with very extensive plexiform neurofibroma involvement has offered hope in rare cases where people have very severe disease and are unable to function in society.[3]

Cutaneous and Subcutaneous Neurofibromas

Wollkenstein and colleagues assessed the impact of disease severity and visibility of NF1 on quality of life using the Short Form 36 Health Survey (SF-36) and questionnaire specific for skin disease.[4,5] The SF-36 contains 32 questions and is a general measure of physical and mental well-being, rather than a disease-specific assessment.[5] The authors found that fears about the development of cosmetic problems had a significant effect on patients' perception of their disease severity, and individuals with prominent visible manifestations suffered from significant emotional disability.[4]

The development of neurofibromas during adolescence is a particular source of distress at a time when teenagers are coping with the familiar issues of self-esteem, self-image, and identity within society. Many feel different from other young people and comment on the thoughtlessness of their peer group and find it difficult to deal with curious and sometimes unfeeling attitudes from strangers.

"I think probably from puberty things changed for the worse … suddenly people started to comment on some of the marks and lumps on my body, people can be so cruel, especially teenagers. I was bullied on and off through school and always felt like the odd one out and didn't belong or fit in. I did start to withdraw a little and found it hard to be accepted for who I was. I always felt different and would always try to hide myself away, and never thought I was good enough, because I had NF1. I couldn't wait to leave school, so that's what I did at age 16 years. I thought that things would be so much better outside of school and all the questions, sniggering and bullying would stop" (retrospective view of adolescence from Mr. Jeremy Meechan).

Individuals express anxiety about the inability to predict the extent and numbers neurofibromas that will develop and this is compounded in some cases by having an older family member with NF1 and a large lesion load. Teenagers and young adults are concerned about social activities such as dancing and swimming when they may reveal cutaneous neurofibromas on the limbs and trunk, usually hidden by clothing. There is disquiet about whether a partner or spouse will cope with increasing skin lesions and changing appearance. Older patients often feel withdrawn and isolated and some make a conscious decision to remain single because of cosmetic problems. One lady recounted that she had been asked to get off a bus as the driver feared that she had smallpox and was infectious.

An individual's self-perception does not always concur with outsiders' views about his or her appearance. Some patients have barely perceptible neurofibromas yet suffer anxiety and depression because of a lack of self-esteem and regard themselves as unattractive. Other people cope extremely well with large numbers of neurofibromas by managing the difficult task of transmitting a feeling of self-confidence and are often helped by supportive family members. One patient stated that she strives to be well dressed and groomed, to style her hair fashionably and to maintain good eye contact when answering questions from strangers about her neurofibromas.

Education

Patients are concerned that they should be given age appropriate and updated information about their condition by clinicians and nurses who are conversant with current diagnosis and management. Several people with skin manifestations of NF1 have been told that there is no need to worry or to have any specific surveillance, and subsequently have produced a child with NF1 and serious complications. Written information containing complex medical terminology may be confusing and provoke unnecessary anxiety, and written and verbal information should be tailored to the needs of the individual. Nurse-led support groups for parents of small children with NF1 may be beneficial in this regard. The positive effect of acquiring knowledge from his parents about a serious complication of NF1 is stated eloquently by a young GSTT patient.

> My name is Jordan and I am nearly eleven years old. I was diagnosed with NF1 when I was nearly three years old. I have a tumour on my optic nerves which means my sight is quite poor. When I was younger I didn't realise what was happening, but gradually my parents explained about NF1 and now I understand what it is. I have lots of ambitions and one was to go up in a helicopter which I did last year in Ireland. I get lots of books in Braille which I really enjoy reading and even though I can't see well I love drawing. NF1 no longer scares me because I am used to knowing that I have it and I just get on with my life.

Neurofibromatosis 2

Factors causing negative impact on quality of life such as, severe hearing loss, balance impairment, facial nerve palsy, visual loss, reduced mobility, and social and emotional problems have been identified as potential psychological burdens in NF2.[6,7] People who are profoundly deaf may rely on lip reading, or depend on relatives or computers to facilitate communication. Facial nerve palsy may compound the problem by impairing quality of speech production and limiting facial expression of emotion as well as causing disfigurement.[7] Fatigue is a common complaint due to the effort required to communicate, particularly in crowded places, and social withdrawal is a frequent consequence.[7] Individuals with balance disturbance have been embarrassed when wrongly perceived as drunk and consequently have limited their social interaction. Loss of mobility resulting from weakness or incoordination causes difficulties in traveling on public transport and patients rely increasingly on relatives or carers. Individuals with NF2 have expressed frustration that local support is lacking due to lack of knowledge about the disease amongst doctors, nurses therapists, and employers.

Measures of Quality of Life in NF2

The preliminary clinical trials of the antiangiogenic drug bevacuzimab to reduce NF2 vestibular schwannomas growth (see Chap. 2 on NF2) have underlined the need for objective measures of quality of life in people with NF2.[8] Neary et al.[5,9] used a detailed postal questionnaire in combination with the SF-36 to identify the extent and severity of quality of life issues in 62 NF2 patients. They found that difficulties with social communication and balance were the major problems for people with NF2. Hornigold and colleagues at Guy's and St. Thomas' NHS Foundation Trust have developed the NFTI-QOL (NF2 impact quality of life) as a specific questionnaire for NF2. It takes 3 min to complete, is easy to score, and comprises eight items including hearing, dizziness and balance, facial palsy, sight, mobility, role and outlook on life, pain, anxiety, and depression (Rachel Hornigold et al., personal communication). Balance was the most frequent problem cited by 50 patients and now many carry an NF2 information card in public settings to increase public awareness and understanding (Rachel Hornigold et al., personal communication). It is likely that the most informative view of the impact of patient-perceived QOL will be dependent on both general measures as well as specific function-based questionnaires.

Hearing Rehabilitation

Patients who are profoundly deaf are prone to anxiety and depression due to social isolation. The Hearing Concern charity LINK in England offers intensive rehabilitation to deafened people and their families and helps them with lip reading, emotional support, and employment. Cochlear implants may provide useful in hearing in individuals with an intact cochlear nerve, and an auditory brainstem implant aids lip reading and the appreciation of environmental sound[10,11] (see chapter on NF2).

"Many NF2 sufferers lose all their hearing – I am no different. I was devastated to learn that I would never hear my mum's voice or listen to my favourite song again, but the most frightening prospect was the isolation and social distance that deafness inevitably brings. After successful surgery at King's College London, to implant the auditory brainstem implant (ABI) I had to wait six weeks before it was turned on – those six weeks were essentially the worst six weeks of my life. It was the first time I had ever experienced complete silence. I felt so vulnerable, conversations were so trivial, but most importantly I felt completely cut off from the world I was living in. The initial feedback from the ABI was a shock; I won't lie to you, the sensations and awareness it gave me were extremely primitive and if anything it was detrimental to lip reading. The first two months were frustrating as my

body was becoming accustomed to a new sense, as that is
what ABI is essentially. However, thanks to my medical team
my supportive family and my own hard work I gradually
understood the sounds that I was hearing. When I combined
quick thinking, analysis and context I was able to interpret
these beeps and buzzes into meaningful conversation. The
sound of ABI is unique to the individual user and for me it
sounds like I am hearing things as if my head is under water.
Everything sounds distorted because the clarity isn't there
but nevertheless I hear sounds which give me awareness that
I thought I would never experience again. It also greatly aids
lip reading and my friends and family will vouch for this. I
have met others who have been less successful with the ABI,
which is why I believe that the tedious, frustrating hard work
at the beginning is essential and completely worthwhile. My
attitude was very much that this is my last chance to "stay in
the hearing world" and achieve goals that I had set previously. Consequently I knew if I didn't put 100% effort and
commitment into the ABI, then I might have regrets and be
left forever wondering what if... Aesthetically it isn't the
most pleasing thing to look at; however, the benefit it gives
me is so great that vanity doesn't come into consideration.
The ABI has surpassed all expectations and has made deafness much less of an issue. I am at university and living inde-
pendently, NF2 may have taken my hearing but it has not
taken my quality of life (personal communication from
Tristan Gray who attends Guy's and St. Thomas' NHS
Foundation Trust NF2 clinic).

Specialist Neurofibromatosis Nurses and Specialist Advisers

The nationally commissioned NF1 and NF2 services in
England have funded neurofibromatosis nurses to provide
psychological support and advocacy for patients. Specialist
neurofibromatosis advisers funded jointly by the Neuro
Foundation (formerly the Neurofibromatosis Association)

and local Hospital Trusts in different areas of the UK, have a nursing or social work background. The role of the neurofibromatosis nurse and specialist adviser varies in each center but usually they attend clinics, provide emotional support and education about NF. Telephone and email advice is accessible for patients and their families. The nurse acts as a link between clinicians in the specialist center and the local area as well as collating information for therapists, schools, and employers. In some centers, transitional services support young people through the difficult period of adolescence and aim to improve self-esteem and independence. Parents groups are arranged by the nurses and meet to provide mutual support and to discuss common issues including difficulties with behavior and schooling. A social network for people aged over 45 years lessens the impact of social isolation and encourages discussion about medical problems.

The Neuro Foundation

This is a lay organization that raises funds to benefit people with NF1 and NF2. Practical and emotional support is given to patients and their relatives and they are advised about local resources and available expert medical help, either locally or nationally. The Foundation produces information leaflets that enable patients to understand their disease and to make the appropriate decisions about surveillance and management.

The Patient as Educator

Much emphasis is placed on the physician as the person who understands the impact of disease on quality of life. The two following inspirational accounts emphasize the resilience, determination, and bravery of the individual in combating serious illness and coming to terms with having neurofibromatosis.

As medical professionals we cannot underestimate the importance of listening to our patients and learning from their experience and wisdom. "I was diagnosed with Neurofibromatosis Type 1 before I could walk. My diagnosis was not a surprise given the fact that my mother had previously been diagnosed with the condition. My childhood was happy and whilst I understood that I had a medical condition, it did not give me cause for concern. For me it was something I "had", in the way other children had freckles. I was never made to feel unusual or special to have it. However, I must admit that I was an unusual child in that I actively enjoyed school and learning. My condition was not hidden from me, I knew from an early age that I would require reconstructive surgery on my face—I had been born with a plexiform neurofibroma on the left side of my face. Moreover, I flatter myself by saying that even at that early age, I understood that this would entail a hospital visit, an operation and horror of all horror's an injection! My entry to the teen world was not heralded by my first real boyfriend, nor by my first disco. Instead, my teens started with the discovery of an optic glioma and a craniotomy on the horizon. I spent the summer recovering, reading and like most girls my age taking an activity interest in the world of fashion and shopping. The following summer I had the first of four reconstructive surgeries in the UK under the care of the excellent maxillofacial surgeon. That September, I started the Irish equivalent of the GSCE's, but three months later my life changed. It was discovered that my optic glioma which had previously remained stable had started to grow and was now affecting the eye-sight in my right eye. The result was an unwanted, unasked for Christmas present of fourteen months of chemotherapy. I won't lie, it wasn't pleasant, I used to dread going down to the hospital to get the treatment as I knew that the next few hours and days would be horrid. But do not get the wrong idea of those 14 months, it was not 14 months of hell on earth, yes there were dark moments but there were also bright moments, the bright moments outshone the dark ones. Although the chemotherapy failed to shrink the optic glioma it succeeded in preventing it from growing further and since 2004 it has remained stable. Yes, the optic glioma has resulted in the near complete loss of sight in my right eye, but you will see me driving on our roads in Ireland (admittedly badly-but then that is not my eyesight I'm just a bad driver!) in my little blue Toyota Yaris. Yes the optic glioma means that I find reading for long periods tiring and headache inducing but there is always and I mean always a solution. Now I listen to audio books on my iPod and my collection ranges from Harry Potter, to Shakespeare and Charles Dickens. I restarted college in 2007, my first year was filled with many new and wonderful experiences from meeting new friends, to learning how to cook for myself, to cramming sessions in the library, to all day spent shopping, to doing my laundry and either not shrinking anything or turning my favourite white shirt pink! The highlight of my second year was been awarded an academic scholarship based on my grades. Last year I completed my penultimate year and achieved a First in my annual exams for and honours degree in Business & Economics. My intention is to complete a master's in Finance and quite possibly a doctorate. NF1 will not stop you achieving your dreams; I will not lie it may make them harder to achieve but then you will savour the achievement all the more" (personal communication from Aoife Quinn).

"I'm now 39, and have learnt that I am no different from anyone else and I deserve the same chances and respect as anyone else with or without NF. I am now married have a step son and have a job that I really enjoy. For many years I thought that my NF was to blame for many things, or maybe my own self doubt let me use it as an excuse. I now have the confidence in myself to overcome many hurdles in life that I have had to deal with. I did feel for a long time that NF had kicked me in the teeth. But actually it was the ignorance of Society" (personal communication from Jeremy Meechan).

References

1. Calm KC. Quality of life in cancer patients: an hypothesis. *J Med Ethics*. 1984;10:124-127.
2. Clayton M. *Leonardo da Vinci: The Divine and the Grotesque*. London: Royal Collection Enterprises; 2002.
3. Lantieri L, Meningaud JP, Grimbert P, et al. Repair of the lower and middle parts of the face by composite tissue allotransplantation in a patient with massive plexiform neurofibroma: a 1-year follow-up study. *Lancet*. 2008;372:639-645.
4. Wolkenstein P, Zeller J, Revuz J, et al. Quality of life impairment in neurofibromatosis 1. *Arch Dermatol*. 2001;137:1421-1425.
5. Garratt AM, Ruta DA, Abdalla MI, et al. SF36 health survey questionnaire: An outcome measure suitable for routine use within the NHS? *Br Med J*. 1993;306:1440-1444.
6. Neary WJ, Hillier VF, Flute T, et al. The relationship between patients' perception of the effects of neurofibromatosis type 2 and the domains of the Short Form-36. *Clin Otolaryngol*. 2010;35:291-299.
7. Patel C, Ferner R, Grunfeld E. A qualitative study of the impact of living with neurofibromatosis type 2. *Psychol Health Med*. 2011;16:19-28.
8. Plotkin SR, Stemmer-Rachamimov AO, Barker FG. Hearing improvement after bevacizumab in patients with neurofibromatosis type 2. *N Engl J Med*. 2009;361:358-367.
9. Neary WJ, Hillier VF, Flute T, et al. Use of a closed set questionnaire to measure primary and secondary effects of neurofibromatosis type 2. *J Laryngol Otol*. 2010;124:720-728.
10. Lusitg LR, Yeagle J, Driscoll CL, et al. Cochlear implantation in patients with neurofibromatosis type 2 and bilateral vestibular schwannoma. *Otol Neurotol*. 2006;27:512-518.
11. Kanowitz SJ, Sahpiro WH, Golfinos JG, et al. Auditory brainstem implantation in patients with neurofibromatosis type 2. *Laryngoscope*. 2004;114:2135-2146.

Chapter 5
Clinical Quiz: Diagnostic and Management Pitfalls of Neurocutaneous Disease

Rosalie E. Ferner, D. Gareth R. Evans, and Susan M. Huson

Quiz Questions

1. A child age 10 years presents with two café au lait patches and two skin lumps. What is the differential diagnosis? What investigations would you do?
2. A patient with NF1 complains of severe pain in one of his fingers if it is knocked. Pressure on the nail bed causes pain. What is the likely diagnosis? What assessment and management would you carry out?
3. A 40-year-old woman presents with a 3-month history of sudden bilateral hearing loss and headaches. Brain MRI shows bilateral enhancing lesions in the cerebellopontine angle. What is the differential diagnosis?
4. What predicts severe disease in NF2?
5. A woman with no family history of NF2 presents with bilateral vestibular schwannomas aged 50 years? What is the risk of her son having NF2?
6. What is the device in Fig. 5.1? What is it used for?
7. This patient in Fig. 5.2 developed painless wasting and weakness in the thigh muscles when he was a child. What is this called? What type of neurofibromatosis does he have?
8. The nodular plexiform neurofibroma in Fig. 5.3 has grown, become firm, and painful. What should you do?

R.E. Ferner et al., *Neurofibromatoses in Clinical Practice*,
DOI: 10.1007/978-0-85729-629-0_5,
© Springer-Verlag London Limited 2011

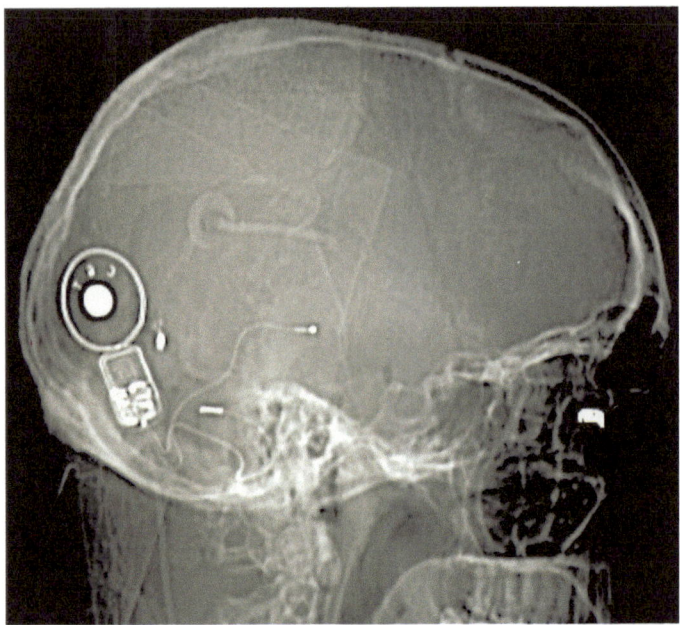

9. A 4-year-old child with NF1 is found to have reduced visual acuity in one eye on routine assessment. The parents think that the child is otherwise well. What would you do?

10. If the cutaneous neurofibromas in Fig. 5.4 cause pain should malignancy be excluded?

11. What abnormalities do you see in Fig. 5.5? What are the symptoms?

12. What is the large lesion in Fig. 5.6 in this patient? What would be the risks in removing it?

13. A 25-year-old woman presents with difficulty walking due to weakness in her legs. On examination she has three café au lait patches, multiple subcutaneous neurofibromas but no cutaneous neurofibromas. She tells you that her father died from complications from a spinal tumor. What kind of neurofibromatosis should be considered?

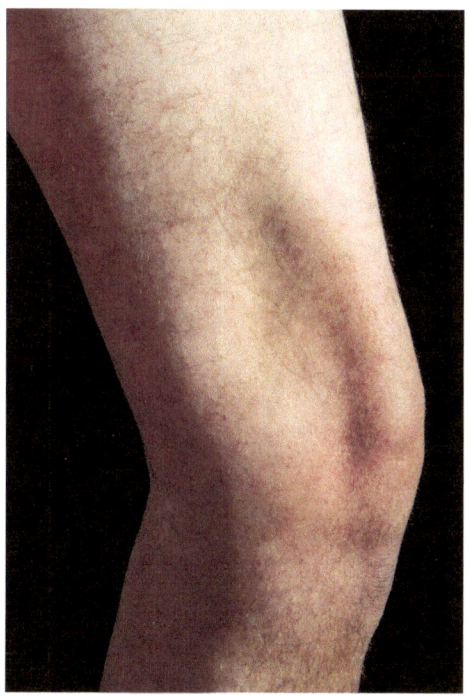

FIGURE 5.2.

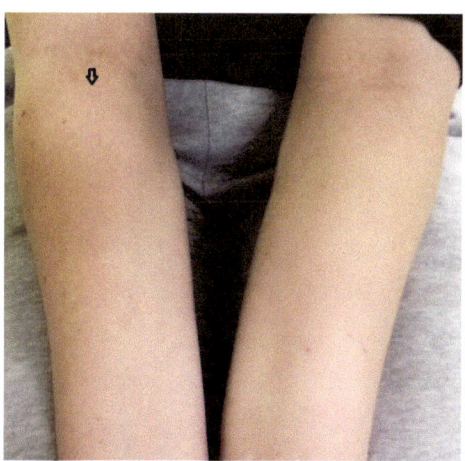

FIGURE 5.3.

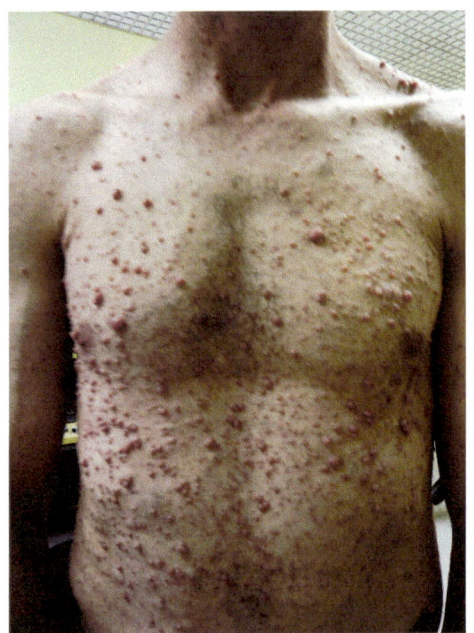

FIGURE 5.4.

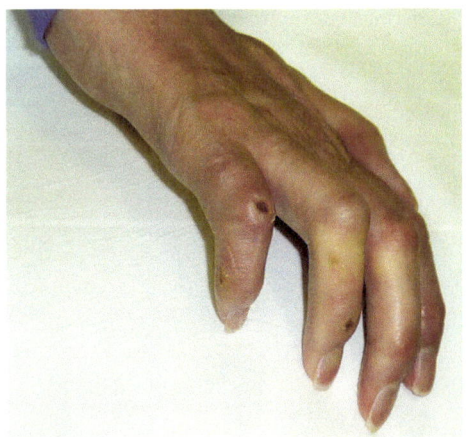

FIGURE 5.5.

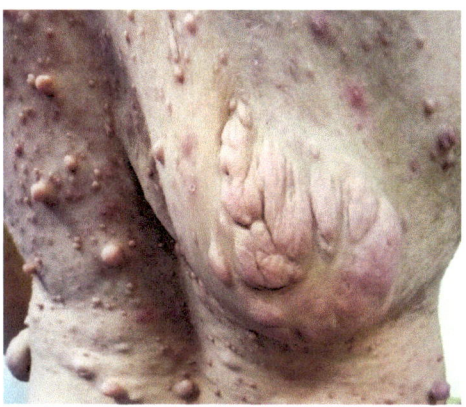

FIGURE 5.6.

14. A 40-year-old woman with uncomplicated NF1 asks for advice about disease monitoring. What would you recommend?

15. A couple with a child with NF1 asks about the risks of NF1 for future children? Should they have prenatal testing?

16. A child with NF1 is having difficulty in concentrating at school. His teachers report that he appears to daydream and frequently loses the thread of a conversation for a couple of seconds at a time. His parents have seen similar behavior at home. What should you do?

17. A woman aged 22 years has NF1 and would like to start on the oral contraceptive pill, but is worried that it might increase neurofibroma growth. What advice would you give her?

Quiz Answers

1. This could be mosaic NF1 or childhood presentation of NF2. Investigations: Full clinical assessment with neurological examination; eye examination to look for Lisch nodules (NF1) or cataracts (NF2). Biopsy of one of the lumps will confirm whether it is a neurofibroma or a schwannoma. (Genetic testing for NF1 if it is a neurofibroma or for NF2 if it is a schwannoma may reveal a mosaic mutation)

2. This is likely to be a glomus tumor. Examination may show a purplish lesion under nail bed and MRI might help locate tumor. Surgical excision will relieve the symptoms.

3. This is a sudden onset of symptoms in an older individual and unusual first presentation for NF2. You must exclude an underlying malignant process such as choroid plexus carcinoma, lymphoma, ependymoma, or melanoma.

4. Early age at first symptom, multiple meningiomas and truncating mutations of the NF2 gene (these are genetic mutations that cause a shortened protein that is often unstable).

5. As the mother presents late in middle age there is a high chance that she has mosaic NF2 so the risk to her son is less than 50%. The risk is 22% prior to molecular testing of the mother and 9% if no mutation is found in the mother. (See Table 2.2, Chap. 2 on Neurofibromatosis 2)

6. This is an auditory brainstem implant for people with profound hearing loss. It stimulates the cochlear nucleus within the brainstem and is beneficial for some patients with NF2. It is inserted when the auditory nerve is absent or is not functioning after tumor surgery. It helps some people with profound deafness to appreciate environmental sound and aids lip reading (Fig. 5.1).

7. This focal wasting and weakness is called amyotrophy and may be the presenting sign of NF2 in childhood (Fig. 5.2).

8. Arrange an urgent assessment by a NF1/MPNST service to exclude malignancy. MRI will show the extent of the lesion and FDG PET CT will assess metabolic activity (Fig. 5.3).

9. Young children do not complain of visual loss. Ensure that a visual assessment including fundoscopy is carried out by an experienced pediatric ophthalmologist. If the visual loss is confirmed, arrange a brain MRI to exclude an optic pathway glioma. Children with optic pathway glioma should be referred to a specialist pediatric oncology team.

10. No, as these lumps are cutaneous neurofibromas and do not become malignant. Pain in a cutaneous neurofibroma may indicate an infection and the patient should be treated with antibiotics. The neurofibroma may be excised once the infection has been treated (Fig. 5.4).

11. Clawing of the hand with wasting of the intrinsic hand mus-
    cles, flattening of the ulnar border, and evidence of injury
    with scars. The patient complained of weakness in the hand
    and loss of sensation for light touch, pain, and temperature.
    She had multiple nerve root schwannomas (Fig. 5.5).
12. This is a diffuse plexiform neurofibroma – note the pur-
    plish hue. Removal would be associated with a risk of
    bleeding and delayed wound healing (Fig. 5.6).
13. Spinal neurofibromatosis. Reasons: This is a rare variant of
    NF1 where multiple neurofibromas on many spinal roots are
    the key feature. There are usually no cutaneous neurofibromas
    but patients may have multiple peripheral nerve lesions.
14. Advise her to ask her clinician if any new or unexplained
    symptoms could be related to NF1? She should have
    annual blood pressure measurement. Women under 50
    years with NF1 have a moderately increased risk of breast
    cancer and she should have annual mammograms and
    then have the same screening regime as the general popu-
    lation. She should seek immediate advice if she develops
    pain, growth, hard texture, or neurological deficit in a
    plexiform or subcutaneous neurofibroma.
15. They should be referred for genetic counseling. In a genetics
    clinic they would be examined to exclude segmental NF1.
    If the examination is normal, the risk of recurrence is much
    less than 1% and prenatal testing is not indicated.
16. He may be having absence seizures. He should be referred
    for an EEG and neurological advice. Absence seizures are
    frequently misdiagnosed as behavioral difficulties in chil-
    dren with NF1. Seizures are reported with increased
    frequency in NF1 and NF2.
17. Neurofibromas increase in size and numbers in pregnancy
    but there is no firm evidence that this happens with oral
    contraceptives. Oral progesterone/progesterone and
    estrogen preparations do not appear to be associated with
    problems. There have been anecdotal reports of increased
    neurofibroma growth in patients receiving high-dose syn-
    thetic progesterone in depot injections. If she is concerned
    she could seek advice about alternative methods of
    contraception.

Appendix

**Rosalie E. Ferner, D. Gareth R. Evans,
and Susan M. Huson**

Useful Addresses

Charities

The Neuro Foundation UK

(The working name of The Neurofibromatosis Association)
Provides support for individuals with NF1 and their families
and information about Neurofibromatosis 1 and 2
Quayside House, 38 High Street, Kingston upon Thames,
Surrey KT1 1HL
Telephone +44 (0)20 8439 1234I
Fax: +44 (0)20 8439 1200I
E-mail: info@nfauk.org
Website www.nfauk.org

Changing Faces

This charity supports people with facial, limb, or body dis-
figurement and their families.
The Squire Centre, 33-37 University Street, London, WC1E
6JN.
Telephone: 0845 4500 275 or 0207 391 9270
Fax: 0845 4500 276
Email: info@changingfaces.org.uk
Website: www.changingfaces.org.uk
Website for young people: www.iface.org.uk

R.E. Ferner et al., *Neurofibromatoses in Clinical Practice*,
DOI: 10.1007/978-0-85729-629-0,
© Springer-Verlag London Limited 2011

Hearing Concern LINK

Supports people with hearing loss and their families and organizes rehabilitation courses
19 Hartfield Road, Eastbourne, East Sussex, BN21 2AR
Telephone: 01323 638230
Text: 01323 739998
Fax: 01323 642968
Web: www.hearingconcernlink.org

Children's Tumour Foundation USA

American Neurofibromatosis Association
Children's Tumour Foundation
95 Pine Street, 16th Floor, New York, NY 10005-4002
Telephone: (00)-1-212-344-6633
Fax: (00) 1-212-747-0004
Email info@ctf.org

Nationally commissioned Neurofibromatosis 1 centres for people with complex NF1

London (Lead Centre)

Guy's and St. Thomas' NHS Foundation Trust
Contact Professor Rosalie E Ferner, Consultant Neurologist
Department of Neurology, Guy's Hospital, Great Maze Pond, London SE1 9RT.

Manchester

Central Manchester University Hospitals Foundation Trust
Contact Dr. Susan Huson, Consultant Clinical Geneticist, Genetic Medicine, 6th floor, St Mary's Hospital, Oxford Road, Manchester M13 9WL.

Nationally commissioned Neurofibromatosis 2 centres

Manchester (Lead centre)

Central Manchester University Hospitals Foundation Trust
Contact Professor Gareth Evans, Consultant Clinical Geneticist, Genetic Medicine, 6th floor, St Mary's Hospital, Oxford Road, Manchester M13 9WL

London

Guy's and St. Thomas' NHS Foundation Trust
Contact Professor Rosalie E Ferner, Consultant Neurologist
Department of Neurology, Guy's Hospital, Great Maze Pond,
London SE1 9RT

Oxford

Oxford Radcliffe Hospitals NHS Trust
Contact Dr Allyson Parry Consultant Neurologist or Dr
Dorothy Halliday
Consultant Geneticist, NF2 Office, Department of Neurology,
West Wing, John Radcliffe Hospital, Headley Way, Headington,
Oxford, OX3 9DU

Cambridge

Cambridge University Hospitals NHS Foundation Trust
Contact Mr Patrick Axon Consultant Skull Base Surgeon,
Skull Base Surgery Unit, Addenbrooke's Hospital, Hills
Road, Cambridge, CB2OQQ

Back Cover Copy

Neurofibromatoses in Clinical Practice provides a succinct,
accessible guide to the neurofibromatoses including diagnosis,
management protocols, and indications for referral to specialist centers. Neurocutaneous diseases are complex to diagnose
and treat and many patients require specialist multidisciplinary
management and surveillance. Due to multiple disease manifestations, patients can present to different clinicians without
specialist expertise such as general practitioners, pediatricians,
neurologists, geneticists, surgeons, and ophthalmologists.

The clinically focused format of this book will enable rapid
consultation during clinics, facilitate disease pattern recognition, and indicate care pathways. The clinical quiz highlights
common pitfalls in diagnosis and management and a glossary
and reference section provide details for access to specialist
NF clinics throughout the UK and internationally.

Written by experts in the field *Neurofibromatoses in
Clinical Practice* is a practical guide for consultants in training
and practice, general practitioners, and specialist nurses.

Glossary of Terms

Amyotrophy Focal wasting and weakness in NF2, particularly involving the small hand muscles or thigh and may be presenting symptom of the disease.

Auditory brainstem implant (ABI) ABI is a device that stimulates the cochlear nucleus within the brainstem. It consists of an external sound processor and an internal electrode that is in contact with the brainstem. It is inserted when the auditory nerve is absent or is not functioning after tumor surgery. It helps some people with profound deafness to appreciate environmental sound and aids lip reading.

Bevacizumab (avastin) Anti-angiogenic drug. Currently used in clinical trial and as treatment in exceptional cases to reduce growth of vestibular schwannomas in NF2.

Bilateral vestibular schwannomas Benign tumors on the eighth cranial nerve that cause hearing and balance disturbance in NF2 patients. Treatment includes surgery, stereotactic radiotherapy (small risk of malignant change), and bevacuzimab in exceptional cases. Sporadic vestibular schwannomas are unilateral and develop in middle age.

Bony dysplasia Abnormalities of bone are due to defective maintenance of bone structure in NF1 patients. Include scoliosis, pseudarthrosis, and vertebral scalloping.

Café au lait patches (also called café au lait spots) Benign skin pigmentation with smooth contours. Six café au lait patches are diagnostic of NF1, but occur in smaller number in NF2. Also seen in patients with Legius syndrome, familial café patches. In the general population 10% may have up to two café au lait patches.

Carcinoid Slow growing neuroendocrine tumor that usually occurs in the duodenum in NF1. May co-exist with pheochromocytoma.

Cardiovascular disease Includes congenital heart disease, especially pulmonary stenosis and hypertension. Associated with NF1.

Cataracts Subcapsular lens opacities. Develop in young people with NF2 and may be presenting feature. Do not usually require treatment.

Cerebrovascular disease Includes stenosis, hemorrhage, and aneurysm of cerebral arteries and occurs with increased frequency in NF1.

Chiari malformation Structural abnormality in cerebellum and brainstem that pushes the brainstem and cerebellum downward. The resulting pressure may cause outflow obstruction of cerebrospinal fluid. Chiari 1 malformation does not usually cause symptoms and is reported in NF1.

Cochlear implant This is a surgically placed electronic device that is placed into the cochlea and stimulates a functioning auditory nerve to produce a sensation of hearing in deaf persons.

Cognitive problems Commonest complication in NF1 and includes low average IQ with specific learning problems and behavioral problems.

Constitutional mismatch repair deficiency syndrome (CMMR-D) This is a recessive condition caused by bi-allelic mutations in one of four mismatch repair genes. Affected individuals have a predisposition to central nervous system, hematological, and bowel malignancy. The phenotype includes multiple café au lait patches and some cases actually have somatic NF1 mutations.

Cutaneous neurofibroma Forms on the skin in people with NF1, always benign and may be purplish in color. Isolated neurofibromas may be sporadic. Cause itching, stinging, and cosmetic problems.

Disfiguring plexiform neurofibroma Large, diffuse neurofibroma of the face, trunk, or limbs that impinges on surrounding structures or is associated with bone hypertrophy. Risks of hemorrhage and delayed wound healing are high.

Dural ectasia Is visible on magnetic resonance imaging as out-pouching of the dura (the outer covering of the spinal cord) and is asymptomatic or occasionally causes pain and neurological deficit in NF1 patients.

Ependymoma Central nervous system tumor arising from ependymal cells and frequently develops in brainstem or spinal cord (particularly upper cervical region) in NF2. Maybe indolent or cause progressive neurological deficit.

Epilepsy Seizures occur with increased frequency in NF1 and NF2, and all seizure types occur. May be associated with tumors or underlying cortical dysplasia

Facial mononeuropathy This may occur in NF2 without an underlying schwannoma and is probably due to Schwann cell proliferation.

Familial café au lait patches In this rare subtype families develop café au lait patches +/– skin fold freckling but do not develop neurofibromas as adults and have a much lower risk of complications. Two genetic causes have so far been identified, SPRED1 mutations (Legius syndrome) and the c.2970-02972 delAAT mutation in the *NF1* gene.

Freckling Benign skin pigmentation under the arms, around the neck, in the groins, diagnostic of NF1.

Gastrointestinal stromal tumor Mesenchymal tumors that may be multiple and usually found in small bowel in NF1. They cause abdominal pain, anemia, or hemorrhage.

Gliomas Arise from the glial or supporting cells of the nervous system, may occur in brain or spinal cord, but mainly involve the brainstem and cerebellum in NF1. Most are low grade but some may behave aggressively. (See also optic pathway gliomas).

Glomus tumor Benign tumor of glomus body which causes exquisite pain in nail bed and may be multiple in NF1 patients.

Legius syndrome This is a milder phenotype than NF1 with café au lait patches, freckling but no neurofibromas and with mutation in the *SPRED1* tumor suppressor gene.

Lisch nodules Benign asymptomatic raised pigmented lesions on the iris, seen on slit lamp examination and diagnostic of NF1.

Malignant peripheral nerve sheath tumor (MPNST) NF1 patients have a 10% lifetime risk of developing MPNST that may be low, intermediate, or high grade. Presentation is with persistent pain, change in texture, rapid increase in size of a lump, or neurological deficit.

Meningiomas Benign tumors that develop in the orbit, brain, and spine, and may be multiple. Characteristic of NF2 but do not occur with increased frequency in NF1.

Merlin (schwannomin) The protein product of the *NF2* gene is related to the moesin, ezrin, radixin, proteins that control growth and cellular remodeling.

Mosaic NF1 The gene mutation (alteration in the genetic message) occurs after fertilization. The proportion of the body affected by the disease is dependent on the timing of the mutation after fertilization. The commonest form is for one body segment to show NF1 skin changes (segmental NF1).

Mosaic NF2 Mosaic NF2 presents as mild generalized NF2 or NF2 features that are localized to one area of the body (e.g., unilateral vestibular schwannomas and meningiomas).

mTOR mTOR mammalian target of rapamycin is involved in cell growth and proliferation. Rapamycin has been used in clinical trials to treat growing plexiform neurofibromas.

Multiple sclerosis Occurs with increased frequency in NF1, particularly primary progressive multiple sclerosis. The clinical manifestations may be confused with symptoms related to optic pathway gliomas or spinal plexiform neurofibromas.

Neuro-cardio-facial-cutaneous syndromes (also called Rasopathies) The collective term given to the conditions caused by mutations in the Ras-MAPK pathway which include NF1 and Legius syndrome.

Neurofibroma Benign peripheral nerve sheath tumor that occurs on or under the skin or on the spinal nerve roots or nerve plexuses. Composed of Schwann cells, fibroblasts, perineurial cells, and axons in an extracellular matrix. (See also cutaneous neurofibroma, subcutaneous neurofibroma, plexiform neurofibroma.)

Neurofibromatosis 1 An inherited neurocutaneous condition that predisposes to benign and malignant tumor formation and is caused by mutations in the *NF1* gene on chromosome 17.

Neurofibromatosis 2 A rare inherited neurocutaneous condition that is characterized by vestibular schwannomas, other benign brain and spine tumors, and cutaneous and eye signs. It is caused by mutations in the *NF2* gene on chromosome 22.

Neurofibromatosis 2 neuropathy Axonal peripheral neuropathy which may be motor and sensory and is progressive in some patients.

Neurofibromatous neuropathy (NF1) An indolent motor and sensory neuropathy in NF1. Affected individuals harbor an increased risk of malignant peripheral nerve sheath tumor.

Neurofibromin The *NF1* gene product is neurofibromin which regulates cell growth and proliferation by inactivation of p21ras and control of mammalian target of rapamycin (MTOR).

NF1 microdeletions This is the genetic mechanism that causes the disease in approximately 5% of people with NF1. In addition to the *NF1* gene the deletion, depending on size, involves a number of other neighboring genes. Microdeletions are associated with more severe clinical manifestations.

Nonossifying fibromas Cystic lesions of bone in NF1 patients that may be painful or cause pathological fracture.

Optic pathway glioma (OPG) These tumors arise from the glial cells in the central nervous system. They form anywhere on the optic pathway but are commonest in the optic nerves in NF1. Most tumors are indolent and do not need treatment, but some cause decreased vision in childhood and require chemotherapy.

Pheochromocytoma Catecholamine secreting tumor, mainly found in the adrenal medulla in NF1. It may be bilateral and is occasionally malignant. It causes hypertension and may coexist with carcinoid tumor.

Plexiform neurofibroma Benign peripheral nerve sheath tumor that grows along the length of the nerve, often involves multiple nerves, frequently causing neurological deficit, and may undergo malignant change in NF1.

Positron emission tomography (PET CT) ([18F]2-fluoro-2-deoxy-D-glucose positron emission tomography computerized tomography) is the optimum way of diagnosing malignant peripheral nerve sheath tumor. It gives qualitative and semi-quantitative evaluation of the metabolic activity of a tumor. It should only be used in NCG specialist centers for this purpose and is not useful for assessing schwannomas.

Preimplantation genetic diagnosis Available for people with NF1 and NF2. Healthy embryos are selected on the third day of fetal development.

Pseudarthrosis Causes bowing of the long bones, most commonly the tibia. Fracture occurs after trivial injury in infancy and childhood with delayed healing. The presentation may be mistaken for nonaccidental injury instead of NF1.

Renal artery stenosis Associated with hypertension in NF1 and caused by dysplasia of blood vessels or aneurysm.

Schwannoma This is a benign nerve sheath tumor composed of Schwann cells and has a capsule. May be sporadic, but multiple lesions are characteristic of NF2 or Schwannomatosis. Malignant change is rare and PET CT does not detect malignant change in schwannomas (see PET CT). In NF2, schwannomas form on cranial, spinal, peripheral, and cutaneous nerves.

Schwannomatosis This rare condition is characterized by multiple schwannomas (but not eighth nerve schwannomas). May be familial, and the gene is tumor suppressor *INI1 (SMARCB1)*.

Scoliosis Curvature of the spine in NF1 that may be idiopathic or dystrophic and the latter may cause neurological or respiratory problems. Occasionally, it may be associated with an underlying plexiform neurofibroma.

Segmental NF1 (see mosaic NF1)

Skin schwannomas Skin schwannomas may be subcutaneous, intradermal, or plaque lesions in NF2.

Sphenoid wing dysplasia Defective formation of the skull bones diagnostic of NF1. The temporal lobe may push forward into the orbit and cause pulsating protrusion of the eye.

Spinal cord compression Spinal nerve root neurofibromas may cause pressure on the nerve roots and spinal cord. Many do not need intervention despite the neuroradiological appearances of cord compression, but some cause neurological deficit, particularly in the upper cervical spine, and require surgery.

Spinal neurofibromatosis Hereditary spinal neurofibromatosis is a rare form of NF1 and the characteristic features are multiple spinal neurofibromas with or without peripheral nerve involvement and relatively few café au lait patches.

Statins Lovastatin reverses ras activity, and statin drugs are being used in clinical trial to treat learning problems in children with NF1.

Subcutaneous neurofibroma This firm, discrete neurofibroma under the skin causes pain and neurological symptoms and may become cancerous.

T2 hyperintensities on brain MRI These are asymptomatic lesions that are found especially in the basal ganglia, cerebellum, and brainstem in people with NF1. They do not cause neurological deficit and disappear with age.

Vertebral scalloping This is pronounced curvature of the dorsal part of the vertebral body and is seen on MRI in NF1 patients and is asymptomatic.

Xanthogranuloma Yellowish nodule occurring transiently on the head, limbs, and trunk in NF1 children.

Index

R.E. Ferner et al., *Neurofibromatoses in Clinical Practice*,
DOI: 10.1007/978-0-85729-629-0,
© Springer-Verlag London Limited 2011